MW00814932

A Serendipitous Life

To DR SMITH —
THANK YOU FOR THE
GREAT C   E LAST
YEARS.'   EN
A BLE

          OOD
     DESIGN+ART

A *Serendipitous* Life

From German POW to American Psychiatrist

Karl Rickels, M.D.

Notting Hill Press

A Serendipitous Life: From German POW to American Psychiatrist
Published by Notting Hill Press
A Division of Winston-Crown Publishing House, Ltd.
PO Box 651
Evergreen, CO 80437
U.S.A.
Phone: 303-674-6304
info@winstoncrown.com
www.winstoncrown.com

Copyright © 2011 by Karl Rickels, MD

Library of Congress Control Number: 2011906540

Cover design by Linda Wood at woodartstudio@bellsouth.net
Cover Photo: © Robert H. Clink
©iStockphoto.com/Dietmar Klement
Editor: Stephen Parolini at www.spwriter.com

All rights reserved. No part of this book may be reproduced or transmitted in any form or by any means, electronic, photocopy, recording or mechanical, without permission in writing from the publisher.

ISBN 978-1-61137-003-4

10 9 8 7 6 5 4 3 2 1

Acknowledgements

I would like to thank my children, Laurence, Stephen and Michael, and my daughter-in-law, Alyssa, for their support and encouragement throughout the process of writing my memoirs. Without their love, helpful suggestions, and gentle pushing, this contribution would not have taken shape into the form it is now. A particular thank you to Heidi, my other daughter-in-law, for her tremendous help in guiding the editing and design work of this book.

Contents

Dedication

This little book is written for you, my grandchildren. And while it was largely inspired by the eldest, Andrew and Peter, it is also written for you, Caroline, Claudia, and Aiden. I had many occasions to spend with Andrew and Peter, searching for *Regenwuermer* by the creek in the woods behind our house; going for long hikes on Gladwyne's bridle path through the "enchanted forest" searching for foxes, wolves, dragons, and for *Hexen* dancing on brooms at midnight; fighting battles with knights and dragons in our house; or going for a trip to the Strasburg steam engine and Dutch Wonderland. I realize how many similar things I had done with your fathers, and Uncle Larry, when they were your age, and how these experiences reminded me of my own childhood.

This prompted me to write down some of my memories. I was further encouraged to write not only about my childhood, but also about my experiences as a young man, as a German soldier and American prisoner of war, as a medical student in post-World War II Germany, and as an immigrant. I was inspired to record the stories of my life when I accompanied you to Shelly Ridge, when I spent time with you in preschool, or had the chance to share with your whole class about German Christmas and my experience as a German immigrant. I still see the wide-open eyes of you and your classmates spellbound by what the old man you call *Opa* was sharing. These wonderful experiences were the final determining events to make me sit down and record what little I remembered of my growing up.

Your Opa has always been an optimist, a person who remembers the good things and forgets, or represses, the bad things. Thus, many of the bad things I experienced, and the poor decisions I made, may not appear in this book. My father, your great-grandfather, used to say to me, "Son, remember and focus only on the positive in life. Do not dwell on the negative, yet learn from it, and always trust the Lord to guide you." This taught me to roll with the punches and not to be afraid to make decisions, nor to be afraid to make mistakes. And believe me, your Opa has made his share of mistakes. As a great man once said, "When you are faced with a decision, the best thing is to do the right thing, the next best thing is to do the wrong thing, and the worst thing is to do nothing."

Grandchildren, I'd like to share one more morsel of wisdom with you, just as your great-grandfather did with me and my sister, your great-aunt, Gisela, and as I did with my sons: "When you're an adult, make it your goal to find a job or profession that you truly enjoy."

I am now in my mid-eighties and you might well ask me why I am still working at the university. The answer is simple: I like what I am doing. It is not only my work but also my hobby. Linda, your Nana, fully supported me in the pursuit of my work and happiness. Bismarck, the German chancellor, who, after the Franco-German war of 1871 was the first in the world to introduce Social Security for old age and universal health insurance, had this Latin phrase on his desk: *Ora et labora,* which, translated, means "pray and work." This reminds me of two German sayings, *Sich regen bringt Segen,* or in English, "Work brings happiness," and *Die Arbeit macht das Leben,* or in English, "Work makes life worthwhile." This is wisdom worth heeding.

When I started to write this book, I became glaringly aware that neither my father nor I had shared much about our pasts. My father rarely talked about his experiences as a German soldier during World War I on the Western front or about his life before the war.

The same is true for *Oma,* my mother. This may have been partially because as children we had little interest in the past; we were much more interested in the present.

But the past has so much to tell us! For example, my father's ancestors on his mother's side can be traced back to the Reformation in the fifteenth century, to a man who was a friend of Martin Luther. In fact, all my ancestors on my father's maternal side were Lutheran ministers. My father's ancestors on his father's side have been traced back four centuries, when, as farmers, they fought suppression by the kings of Denmark and created their own Lutheran farmer state in the sixteenth century.

On my mother's side there were six generations of farmers and small business people, all Roman Catholic. My father, the Lutheran, and my mother, the Catholic, raised three children as Catholics, in the mother's faith, as was customary at the time. My father went weekly with us to the Catholic church, but he remained a Lutheran.

And look at Nana's ancestors. Nana's mother, Nana Bee, your great-grandmother, was the descendent of William Bradford, who came to Plymouth in Massachusetts on the Mayflower in 1620, and was for many years the governor of the new colony. The ancestors of Papa Joe, Nana's father and your great-grandfather, can be traced back to before the Declaration of Independence. Because of this ancestry, you all are descendents of the Mayflower, and all could join this astute organization to which your great-grandmother, Nana Bee, belonged. Since your great-grandmother also belonged to the Daughters of the American Revolution, Caroline and Claudia could also join this organization, while you boys could join the Sons of the American Revolution.

I grew up in Germany during the Depression. In America, President Roosevelt wasn't yet in power. I was eight years old when the

Nazis came to power. I became a prisoner of war and was in America when Roosevelt died in 1945 and President Truman succeeded him. Truman was a strong decision maker. The "little man" from Kansas was a real man, not afraid of his new job. In fact, Truman decided to drop the atomic bomb on Japan, thus ending World War II and saving thousands and thousands of US soldier's lives. I still remember something from that time that really impressed me. Mr. Hopkins, President Roosevelt's secretary, came to Truman's office and told him, "Mr. Vice President, the president has died," to which Truman responded, "The president is not dead, I am the president."

All the news in those days we learned either from the radio or the newspaper. TV and tape recordings did not yet exist, and of course there were no CDs, video games, or computers. For entertainment, we read books or played with our friends. Oh, we also had movies, but nothing like you have today.

And this is just the tip of the iceberg. There is so much to be learned from looking back.

One final note: Germans like to create long sentences and put the verb at the very end. Sometimes while reading this book you might feel as if you are on a treasure hunt searching for the verb of the sentence, I hope you will bear with me and keep reading.

—YOUR OPA

1

Growing Up in Germany

As was the case with most Berliners at that time, I was not born in Berlin. I was born on August 17, 1924, in Wilhelmshaven, a large navy town on the North Sea known for its military ship-building and as a navy port. When I was two years old, my parents moved with me from Wilhelmshaven to Berlin. For four years we rented the second floor of a house on the Oranke Lake in Berlin-Hohen-schoenhausen, across from a protected beach. The owner of the house had a large Saint Bernard with whom I frequently played. I remember walking home from the lake for lunch, a white sheet hanging on the balcony was my signal that lunch was ready. Since I was no more than four or five years old at the time, this speaks to the safety and the village character in this part of Berlin.

My father, whom I called *Vati,* Karl Eduard Rickels, was born in Sande, Ost Friesland, in northern Germany, on August 7, 1895. He attended school in Wilhelmshaven, and after the tenth grade he entered a mid-level training program of the postal service. His father died of tuberculosis before I was born. His mother lived until the age of ninety-two in Sande, still tilling the garden, cooking, and doing housework until her death. She died of a respiratory infection because she stubbornly refused to take her prescribed sulfa medication. She complained that it upset her stomach.

My father had four brothers. One, whom I never met, died early of tuberculosis. Georg, the oldest, owned a wholesale candy business in Sande. The second oldest was Fritz, who was less than two years older than my father. Uncle Fritz and my father were both volunteers in World War I. My father was wounded, but he never talked about his time as a German soldier.

I recently learned from my sister, Gisela, that Vati volunteered for the army at the onset of World War I. He was assigned to a cavalry unit, and this saved his life. In a moment of serendipity—a theme that would define my own life for many years—he fell off his horse and broke a leg. During the time he was in the hospital, his unit was involved in an attack on the French at the Somne, France, and the whole unit was destroyed. After the war Vati and Uncle Fritz studied at home from books for the German *Abitur,* the equivalent of a high school diploma, and then went to Wilhelmshaven and sat for the Abitur exam.

After the Abitur, Vati and Uncle Fritz moved to Muenster to study economics while continuing to work for the postal service. One semester they both had to study in Goettingen, as a certain course was not offered in Muenster. Vati went to Goettingen twice to take the semester tests, once for himself and once for Uncle Fritz because Fritz had to keep their postal service job occupied. During their studies both my father and Fritz belonged to one of the many political parties existing in the Weimar Republic.

When this particular party joined the southern Nazis, my father left the party and all politics. But Uncle Fritz did not; he remained in the party and soon became the mayor of Greifswald, a Hanse

town on the Baltic that was home to a small university. When Uncle
Fritz had some business in Berlin, he always stayed with us overnight. I remember the heated discussions Vati and Uncle Fritz had
after dinner. They never got loud enough for me to identify the subjects of their arguments, but I assume it had to do with the Nazis.

Both brothers graduated with doctoral degrees in economics.
Around 1922, after graduation, my father took a position at the
steel works in Willich, a small town of fewer than 5,000 in the
Rhineland, near the larger town of Krefeld. My father rented a small
apartment in my mother's house. This is where he met my mother.
They were married in 1923.

My mother, whom I called *Mutti*, was born Stefanie Theodora
Roehrhoff on September 30, 1901, and raised in Willich where she
went to elementary school. She later went to Krefeld to the academic high school from which she graduated with an elementary
teaching degree, though she didn't teach until she was about fifty,
after my father's newly reopened candy factory near Frankfurt went
bankrupt after the war.

My mother's oldest brother, Heinrich, was killed in World War
I, and her younger brother, Richard, trained as a druggist. He had
his drugstore and his photo lab in his parents' home, where he lived
with his sisters, Kaetchen and Hanna. All three of my mother's siblings never married. Aunt Hanna was office manager in a large au-
ditor office in Krefeld and Aunt Kaetchen operated a hardware and
china store, also in the same house. She also took care of the household. My mother had one other sister, Thekla, whom I never met, as
she died of tuberculosis when she was young. I still remember, and
it continues to impress me, that Aunt Kaetchen could catch flies by
just grabbing them out of the air.

All three of my mother's siblings died after I had immigrated into the United States. Aunt Hanna died of a heart attack, caused by damage to her heart from rheumatic fever as a child. Aunt Kaetchen died in her late sixties of a strangulated simple inguinal hernia. She did not go to see a doctor since she had self-diagnosed herself as having cancer. Uncle Richard died under anesthesia for a minor operation in a small town hospital. His heavy drinking might have contributed to his untimely death. He could empty a large stein of beer in one continuous gulp and won many drinking competitions.

Willich was a large farming community, and my mother's father was the blacksmith of Willich. His shop was approved for the training of new blacksmiths. Their house was on the main street and the property ran all the way to the next street behind, where the blacksmith shop was. After the war my aunts kept chickens and a pig in the courtyard between the main house and the former blacksmith shop.

My grandfather was a tall, strong, and well-respected man. For his military duty he served in the special guard unit which protected the German *Kaiser* (emperor) in his castle in Berlin. One might say he served in the forerunner of the present Secret Service.

My mother's parents died when I was very small. I remember only one visit when I must have been three or four. The whole family had sat down to dinner, but I had to excuse myself early to go to bed. Before leaving I said, "goodnight." Then I went to one distant aunt and kissed her. When I was asked why I had kissed her, I answered, "She is so pretty."

My father died in 1971 at age seventy-six after a stroke caused by ten teeth extractions performed at the same time. Prior to the dental surgery, my father was a completely healthy man. He lived for four more months after the surgery and died at home in Eschborn near Frankfurt, at my sister Gisela's house where Vati and

Mutti had the upstairs apartment. Mutti died at home peacefully when she was eighty-nine.

Early Childhood Memories

I don't recall many memories from my youth, but the ones I do remember are good and happy. I recall a day when I was playing in a nearby field with some other children; I do not remember whether they were boys or girls. We had a magnifying glass and we were using it to focus the sunrays on dry leaves and dry branches. Sure enough, we managed to start a little fire. Like so many German children of that time, we were pretending to be American Indians.

Aunt Hanna visited us frequently and she took me on many walks. She told my mother that she always enjoyed being with me, but she wished I would ask fewer questions. Apparently my favorite three words were, "What is this?" I must have been a curious child.

My parents moved from Hohen-Schoenhausen, a rural area, to Berlin-Lichtenberg, shortly before I entered first grade in a Catholic elementary school.

We shared the courtyard with a Lutheran elementary school on the next street. At that time, and even during the Nazi time, Catholic and Lutheran children went to separate state, not private, elementary schools. During the long recess, about twenty minutes once a day, we had to walk in orderly rows in a circle around the courtyard, as directed by a few teachers. This was both for exercise and for control of unruly children. It's interesting to note that during this time, 1930, there were no preschool or even kindergarten classes. Everyone started with the first grade. It speaks for the safety of this part of Berlin, that even as a first grader, I walked alone to school. It was at least a thirty-minute walk.

Our desks were made for two pupils. We had to sit quietly at our seats until called upon, and when we did something wrong or made noise, we'd get a couple strikes with a cane across the hands or on our behinds. Fortunately, this didn't happen often to me. We never wrote on loose paper, as is now the case in schools, but only in notebooks, with one notebook for German, one for math, and so on.

At age ten one could volunteer to go to the Gymnasium—an academic high school meant to prepare students for entering the university. Those who tested well were allowed to transfer. I went to the Real-Gymnasium Lichtenberg, just five minutes from where we lived. Our school was built in 1911 in the Renaissance style. These schools weren't free, so we had to pay a small tuition (which could be forgiven for those whose parents could not afford to pay). After World War II, the Russians closed the building as a school, and by 1950 it had been converted into the Theater An der Parkaue, a children's theater.

The area where I grew up, Lichtenberg, was at that time a sub-urb complete with vegetable farms, and it was located in the eastern sector of Berlin. Lichtenberg had been a separate village but became a part of Berlin when it was annexed before World War I. Most of Lichtenberg, farther north, consisted of tenement houses for factory workers.

Our apartment, Am Stadtpark 12, had its own garage in the basement and fronted a city park. The main hallway led to a Berlin room with a large window to the courtyard. The Berlin room was so named because many Berlin apartment buildings were built around a courtyard and had two entrances, one for the help, and one for the owner. The Berlin room connected the two. On the other side of this room was a sliding door leading into a large formal dining room where we ate all of our meals.

We had several courses, and Else, our maid, would serve each course separately after being called by my mother with a bell located under the carpet below my mother's right foot. The dining room was also connected by a sliding door to the living room, and all rooms, including bedrooms, had a door to the front hallway, or ante room, which featured a couch, two easy chairs, and the *garderobe,* an elegant wooden contraption for coats and hats and gloves and scarves. The front bathroom and my bedroom had windows facing the courtyard.

All ceilings were at least ten feet high, and we had separate central water heat for each apartment. The heater was in the kitchen. Some rooms also had large tile ovens left over from the time when no central heating system existed. From about 1941 on we only had hot water on weekends, in order to save coal. Most of our daily life took place in the living room.

In our apartment complex there were separate storage areas in the attic for each apartment. The laundry, used by all apartments, with its boiler, wrangler, and scrubber, was also located in the attic. Before modern washing machines, laundry, when at all possible, was boiled. The laundry was then hung on lines to dry. Laundry that could not wait to be cleaned for two or three weeks had to be washed by hand in the apartment.

Our coal was stored in the basement. We had to carry this up to the apartment every day. I would have stored my bike in the basement, but I was afraid to go down there alone. I worried I might run into robbers or other bad men. Also, the light in the basement was on a timer and only stayed on a short time. It was always a little scary when the light went off because I had to quickly find the switch in the dark to turn it on again.

Shopping was all done by foot. This meant that shopping was

done daily. Else and Mutti even had to carry the potatoes from the market to our home. We had no pushcarts or other such gadgets at that time, and certainly no supermarkets. However, warm bread rolls and milk were delivered every morning to our apartment. Walking, bicycling, and public transportation were our ways of traveling within Berlin. Walking never harmed anyone.

Since our family had no car, it was always great for me to visit relatives in Willich and Sande. Uncle Max Windhausen, my mother's cousin who lived in Willich, and Uncle Georg, who lived in Sande, had cars. They took us on day trips that we greatly enjoyed. I also enjoyed the eight-hour train ride from Berlin. Steam locomotives pulled the express trains, and I would stand for hours at an open window, feeling the rush of air, and sometimes also small pieces of coal, blowing in my face.

At the corner between Am Stadtpark and Kielholz Strasse was a fountain and a roundabout where my friends and I held our bike races. Our school was located at one end of our street, surrounded by the park. In the park was a large hill bordering Berlin's largest freight switching yards. In the winter this hill became the sledding hill of Lichtenberg. In the middle of the park was a *Flieder Allee* (lilac walk), where the branches reached from one side of the path to the other. There also was a large children's playground, including sandboxes for children to play in while their mothers or nannies sat on the surrounding benches, happily lost in conversation. There also was a small lake surrounding a small island. Ducks and swans nested there.

An apple farm was conveniently located right next to our apartment building, and we boys liked to climb over the stone wall to eat, or should I say steal, an apple. Sometimes we were chased away, but these apples tasted so much better than the ones we had at home that it was worth the risk.

I was certain then, and am still convinced today, that I grew up in one of the best places in Lichtenberg.

When I was still quite small, I belonged to a clique (Berliners liked English words). I was always the youngest and thus somewhat protected by the other members of the group. It must have been a forerunner of present-day gangs, although much less violent. Often children from other neighborhood streets would invade our territory, which bordered on the city park. We armed ourselves with slingshots to chase them away. The big chestnut trees were our protection year-round and our source of ammunition in the fall, when chestnuts replaced small stones in our slingshots.

As kids we always visited the annual auto show. It was exciting to see all the racecars from Mercedes, Audi, Bugatti, and Maserati. The same cars would race yearly on the Avus, the famous Berlin racetrack. I still remember the 1937 Mercedes sport car that the father of one of my friends owned. (I also remember that the father owned a sauerkraut factory. Sauerkraut must have been a lucrative business then.) The car had eight turbochargers, and four big metal silver hoses on each side of the engine. All the boys in our little group admired it.

I spent all my free time outside with my scooter, and later with my bike. We played marbles on the earth around the trees. We also played *Triesel* (Spin Top), a game in which we would drive a cone-shaped object across the asphalt-lined street with a whip made out of a stick and cord. All children also liked hopscotch. We played soccer wherever we happened to be. We could always freely play on the street because it was rarely traveled by cars. And yet, once, when I was seven or eight, I was run over by a motorbike. I still have the scar over my right eye. At that time people would not go for such little things to an emergency ward, so I was taken to our local doctor who clamped the wound with a few clips.

But much to my regret during those early years, I had to come home early every evening, earlier than my friends, it seemed. My father believed that the sleep before midnight was the healthiest for small children. And every night after I got ready for bed I always had to show my mother or father that I had brushed my teeth. They always checked.

We children also liked to ice skate in the winter. When it was cold enough we walked through gardens and to a restaurant that owned a lake on the Herzbergstr. There we could skate and play hockey. To warm up, we would drink hot apple juice in the restaurant. When it wasn't cold enough for the lake to freeze, we took a streetcar to Friedrichshain, a city park with an artificial ice skating rink. In my young teen years I belonged to an ice hockey club there. Our winters were usually quite snowy from December until the end of February. That's when we enjoyed the sledding hill of Lichtenberg.

In the summer we children also loved to swim and to get a nice tan. We did not belong to a private club, but used the public swimming pools. We even had beaches on either the Wannsee Lake in the West or on the Mueggelsee Lake in the East. After the 1936 Olympic games in Berlin we also could use the Olympic swim stadium. But mostly Vati took us after work to the Spree River in Treptow, only two stations away by the elevated train. The bathing facilities were right in the Spree.

A Shift in the Political Wind

I was eight years old when the Nazis came to power. My parents didn't discuss politics at home. What I remember about that time, both before the Nazis came to power and afterwards, was that Germany was in a similar depression as the United States. Millions of people were jobless. In Berlin, the Communists, particularly in the East where we lived, were very powerful. Fights between Communists and Nazis occurred frequently in the tenement area of Lichtenberg. Every day hungry, jobless people (mostly men) would come to our door. Mutti or Else, our maid, would make them sandwiches or give them a little money. Stealing and burglary became common during this time. Our apartment door had three locks, metal bars, and a peephole. My stroller, and later my bike, had to be carried into the apartment and kept in our back hallway next to the kitchen. Everything had to be double and triple locked.

Our apartment was on the first floor, just one flight up. There were no elevators, as the apartment house had only three floors plus an attic. The apartment had two entrances, front and rear. The rear entrance, used by our maid, was accessed via the *Hof*, the courtyard, which was surrounded on four sides by apartments. The courtyard was visited by all kinds of people, including the knife and scissor sharpener and the music man with a small monkey on his shoulder, who expected us to throw small coins wrapped in paper down out of the window in appreciation for his music.

The *Hinterhaus* was the row of apartments along the back of the courtyard. This is where some of the people lived who worked for the owner of the apartment block. After the Nazis started persecuting Jews, the Jewish owner of our apartment complex moved from her elegant apartment in the front to one in the Hinterhaus, where she was more or less hidden from the police. She stayed there during the war. When the Nazis stopped the family from going into the air raid shelter in the basement, other renters opened a special shelter for them so that they could find protection from the air raids. They were still living there when I left for Africa, and my parents told me later that everyone else in the Hinterhaus later hid them so they never had to go to a concentration camp. And though the front apartments where my parents lived were bombed out, the Hinterhaus was not.

I recently read a book by Albert Speer, who, as a young man, was Hitler's architect and belonged to his inner circle of friends. Speer was never part of the top policy makers, but during the war he became the minister responsible for road rebuilding and armament. After World War II, the International Military Tribunal tried him in Nuremberg, along with other Nazis. Speer was sentenced at the Nuremberg Trials of 1947 or 1948 to twenty years in the Spandau Prison outside of Berlin. He wrote two books during that time. They were written on toilet paper and smuggled out of prison. These books supported my vague memories and impressions of that time. My aunt Kaetchen told me after the war that the only "deadly sin" she ever committed in her whole life happened in Berlin one Sunday morning at election time. She went to the polling place and it was full of brown shirts and SS, scaring her so much that she voted for Hitler.

I remember vaguely that certain foods and materials were in short supply even before the war. We had to collect toothpaste and shaving cream tubes when they were empty because of their precious metal content. The Nazis also promised their people the Volkswagen (VW), yet the only VWs built were for the military. However, the Nazis built a few passenger ships for the working class. They called the organization *Kraft durch Freude* (strength through happiness). These cruise ships were the first cruise ships built, taking the name from the Crusades of the tenth and eleventh century.

When Hitler's Nazi party came to power in 1933, they obtained only 44 percent of the total vote, but it was the largest of eight to ten parties. In Berlin the Nazis only obtained 22 percent of the vote. Berliners were mostly Social Democrats and Communists. The mass rallies in Berlin, Nuremberg, and other cities were staged with a minority of Germans. By 1937, Hitler, who initially attracted excitement, had lost his ability to draw crowds. When he appeared somewhere unannounced, no one came to cheer him. Everything was staged. Since my parents stayed away from politics, I never saw Hitler personally. From age ten to fourteen, I belonged to the *Jungvolk,* or young folk, the equivalent of the Boy Scouts. We were too young to have to march at the Nazi rallies. Only the Hitler Youth, who were fourteen to eighteen years old, had to march.

Yet, in a dictatorship, the government could easily sequester bad events. Remember there was no TV, only radio and newsreels in the movie theaters. There were rumors about concentration camps for people who opposed the party, but never about the killings that were going on. And many of the apolitical Germans buried their heads in the ground and just didn't want to hear about any of it. They said, "This could not be true."

The joblessness in Germany, which partially brought the Nazis to power, now disappeared, and young, unemployed men found jobs on public work projects before being drafted into the army. *Kristal Nacht* happened in 1938, when synagogues were burned and Jewish store windows broken. This event was upsetting for the majority of Germans, including our acquaintances who were Nazis. Beginning in 1937, all scarce material was collected and used for weapons. Very few people could travel outside of Germany because it was almost impossible to obtain foreign currency.

High School Adventures

In the Gymnasium, or high school, which included the fifth through twelfth grades, people from all religions—Protestants, Catholics, and Jewish alike—all studied together. Mine was a boys-only school and the girls had their own high school, which was called a *Lyceum*. We started learning French in the fifth grade, Latin in seventh grade, and English in ninth grade. We continued with Latin and English until the twelfth grade, but could drop French after grade nine to select a natural science track, which I did. I already knew at that time that I wanted to become a physician. When we had to write about what we wanted to be when we were grown, I wrote "a surgeon," but I misspelled the German word. When my teacher checked my story he said to me, "Rickels, if you want to become a surgeon, don't you think you should know how to spell the word?" Needless to say, I was very embarrassed.

Once we started with a subject, we had this subject each year until completing the Gymnasium, but as time went on we had fewer hours per subject than in the first year or two. The teacher's desk and chair stood at the front of the classroom in a podium area one step higher than the classroom. The blackboard was also accessible via the podium. We liked to play jokes on our teachers, like the time we placed white lab mice under the podium. Students were always addressed by their last name, and from tenth grade on, not with the more personal *Du*, but with the more formal *Sie*, as adults addressed each other. We do not have this distinction in the English language.

Children who did not enter the Gymnasium after four years of elementary school would continue in elementary school for four or five more years. After that they would work as apprentices and go to an occupational school part-time for two or three years to learn a trade. For example, many medical technicians who, after the war, worked for my sister, Gisela, had chosen this course of education. Gisela's medical practice was approved for such apprenticeship training. Another option was for children to leave school at the age of 16, after attending the Gymnasium for only six years, instead of graduating with what is called *Abitur*. The Abitur is the prerequisite for entering a university.

My school, which was built into the town park, was a five-minute walk from our house, or three minutes if I ran, which I usually did, since I was always late leaving my home. Each grade had two classes of between thirty and thirty-five students in the early years, and between fifteen and twenty students in the later years. School lasted from eight in the morning to about one thirty in the afternoon, and most of my classes were held in the same room; the teachers came to us. Only physics, chemistry, art, and music were taught in special rooms.

There was no school on Saturday, and teachers were not permitted to give homework over the weekend. After the first two hours of classes we had a long recess of about twenty minutes, when we had to go out into the schoolyard whenever the weather allowed it. Free milk was provided. I almost never had breakfast at home and ate my sandwich during recess. This reminds me of our live-in maid, Else. Part of her job was to make my lunch for school, but she always used too much butter on my sandwiches. Thankfully, my mother discovered this and decided to get up early every day to fix my sandwiches the way I liked them.

In the summer when it got very hot, the school had to let us go home if the temperature was seventy-eight degrees Fahrenheit or above in the classrooms by ten o'clock in the morning. Trying to prevent this from happening, the school workers would water the courtyard, usually to no avail.

School included two hours each week of Physical Education. In the winter we enjoyed activities inside; in the summer, we went outside where we had an area reserved for the broad jump and high jump and for soccer games. We would also run 400, 1500, and 3000-meter races in the adjacent park. I was a long distance runner and ran the 3000-meter.

One day per week in the summer we would have track and field practice, or soccer and handball practice at the Lichtenberg Herzberg Stadium, to which we traveled by streetcar or bike. I played on the school's handball team, at a forward position. Handball is a typical northern European game that is played on a soccer field. As with soccer, handball is played with eleven players per team, and in similar positions to soccer. The ball either had to be dribbled on the ground every three steps, or had to be passed to someone else. The goal was marked by a half circle of chalk over which the forward could not step before throwing the ball toward the goal. Its diameter was, I believe, ten meters. If the ball touched a player's foot, the player was penalized in the same way players are penalized in soccer when they touch the ball with their hands. Our handball team played all over Berlin.

In the winter we did all the gymnastics that are now in the Olympics: double and single bars, horses, rings, and ropes. We also had boxing and wrestling, and always at the beginning of gym class, stretching exercises and push-ups.

For several years I also belonged to the rowing club. We traveled by elevated train to Gruenau on the Spree River where we had our boathouse. It also included an indoor setup for rowing practice in the winter. For two years I also belonged to the school ski club and we traveled by train over Christmas holidays to the mountains separating Czechoslovakia from Germany, sleeping in sleeping bags on the floor of a dairy farmer's house, warmed by the largest tile stove I have ever seen.

For at least two winters in the fifth and sixth grade we would travel to the town's indoor pool one day a week. Every student in the school had to pass a swim test, which meant one had to stay afloat for forty-five minutes in the deep end, swimming or treading water. Many of us also took the lifeguard test.

Our school was the only school in Berlin which owned a *Land-schulheim* (something like a youth hostel or camp) in Tangersdorf, about one hundred kilometers (seventy miles) north of Berlin in the state of Brandenburg. A farmer who lived on the wooded land took care of the property, including setting up bunk beds and an eating area in what used to be a barn. The bunk beds had straw mattresses, and the barn had no heat, but it was the most wonderful place to visit.

During the time that school was in session, one class at a time would enjoy a seven-to-ten-day visit to Tangersdorf. Many students went with the teacher by train and then had to walk a few kilometers to the site. My friends and I always rode our bikes. The first year we rode all one hundred kilometers from home, and all other years we gathered up our knapsacks, loaded our bikes into the cars that had been used for disabled people from World War I, and rode the train to Oranienburg. From there, we rode our bikes the rest of the way (which was still about eighty kilometers).

We usually chose to go during May. The weather at that time was warm, and perfect for swimming in the lake on the property. While there, we still had about two hours of school each day, but we choose often one of our Gym teachers as the chaperone, and so we almost never had classes during our Tangersdorf time. As is typical with boys, after we went to bed, we would tell stories. We also would hold competitions to see who could fart the most. We always had a great time, swimming in the lake, playing ping-pong in the courtyard, and carrying big hunting knives on our belts, with which we practiced knife throwing. And at night we played trapper and Indians in the dark woods. Those students who had no money to go on holiday in the summer with their parents, could go to Tangersdorf for very little money.

Linda and I visited there a few years ago on one of our trips to Berlin. It did not look much different to me then as when I was a student.

All of our teachers had advanced degrees, and most had PhDs. But that didn't stop them from occasionally making us laugh. Our physics teacher was easily distracted. I still remember how he wanted to demonstrate the "time of a free fall of a stone." His plan was to drop a stone from the highest floor to the basement through the stairwell. He held the small stone in one hand and a stopwatch in the other. But instead of pressing the stopwatch and dropping the stone, he pressed the stone and dropped the stopwatch. Our chemistry teacher impressed us by sticking two fingers into liquid sulphur, over 350 degrees Fahrenheit, to demonstrate to our class its liquid consistency.

Just as in the States, at some age level, students went to dancing classes. These were more formal in Berlin than in the United States, when my sons had dancing lessons. They were always held in the western part of the city, in the center of Berlin around the *Tiergarten*. I must have been about thirteen or fourteen years old when I started dancing classes. We had to wear a suit and tie and white gloves when we danced. This kept the sweat from messing up the girls' dresses. Because our family didn't have a car (neither of my parents ever learned to drive), we traveled there like we traveled anywhere else we couldn't get to by bike—by subway or elevated train. I always went with a friend of mine whose parents owned the local bakery. Yet these dancing lessons did not help me to find a girlfriend. I was always somewhat shy.

I took piano lessons from the time I was ten until I was sixteen from Mr. Isleib, who had a studio next to our S-Bahn station. Once a year his students performed before parents and relatives in a concert hall. I hated these piano recitals and, since I never learned to play by ear, I always had to look at the music sheet. But I'm thankful for those lessons. I still play Schubert or Beethoven sonatas from time to time. It's interesting to note that during the war Mr. Isleib talked negatively about the Nazis, attacking them constantly. He didn't hide his feelings. Yet, none of his pupils reported him to the SS, and he continued to give piano lessons until his apartment was bombed in early 1945 and he was killed.

I did a lot of reading when I was a child, particularly Karl May books. Karl May wrote sixty-three books, and I owned most of them and read them several times. Many books focused on the United States and how the whites slaughtered the Indians; the heroes of his Indian books were two trappers, Old Shatterhand and Old Surehand, and the Indian Apache Chief, Winnetou. Yet Karl May was never in the United States. There are still Karl May festivals every summer in Germany.

After my third year in the Gymnasium, at age twelve, my parents received a blue letter. This usually means something official and is rarely good news. However, to my surprise, the letter suggested that I was doing so well in school I should skip the next year, the eighth grade, and go right into the ninth grade. Because of my birthday, August 17, I was one of the oldest in my class, but this was a surprise. My parents accepted, and the whole summer vacation I took lessons to catch up in math and in other fields of study. While I had been an "A" student up until then, when I graduated from high school, I was only a "B" student. We had no "A" students in our graduating class. Lots of missed school time, and the nights frequently spent in air raid shelters due to the war, may have been contributing factors to the lowering of all of our school grades. I believe skipping the eighth grade ultimately worked to my advantage, in fact, most likely saving my life later on.

When I grew up, we listened to the radio and read books because televisions weren't yet widely available or used. But during the summer Olympics in Berlin in 1936, Germany placed one of the early television sets in a large room in the Lichtenberg post office. We went there to watch the Olympic events on TV. However, any news we learned we got from the radio or black and white newsreels at the theater. A movie theater always showed the newsreel first, then American cartoons, and finally the main feature.

Our main movie theater was the *Schwarzer Adler* (black eagle) and there was another at the *Petersburgerstr.* I have forgotten the name. Children also enjoyed visiting the *Schmaler Handtuch* (small hand towel). It was very narrow, less than ten seats wide, and quite deep. We went there for children shows like Mickey Mouse, Laurel and Hardy, and other American films. Laurel and Hardy in the early 1930s made their films first in English and then in several European languages because the method was not yet well developed to synchronize other languages. This was done with all Hollywood films at that time. There is still a great deal of interest in Germany in those old American films. We loved Wild West films the best and frequently played trapper and Indians. We usually pretended to be Indian chiefs wearing a big head gear of feathers and carrying bow and arrows over our shoulders.

On Sundays we went to the Catholic church. In Germany only very few people took communion regularly. While my mother and the children sat in a pew, Vati always stood at the back of the church. One day I asked him why he was not sitting with us. He said, "a Lutheran does not kneel," and it would have been embarrassing for him if he would stand while all others kneeled.

We also had religion as a school subject in the Catholic elementary school and even later in the Gymnasium. During these classes, protestant students had their own religion classes with a teacher while a priest led ours. The Jewish boys had these hours off. Berlin was primarily a protestant town.

Family Dynamics

My mother helped me with language homework in the afternoon— she knew all of the French or English or Latin words that I did not know. That saved me from looking at the dictionary. My father helped with math and physics. I also always liked to prepare for schoolwork that would come up the next day.

My father always came home for dinner (what is typically called lunch in America). This is when we had our main meal of the day. In the evening we had supper, which consisted primarily of sandwiches and warmed-up lunch leftovers. The warmed-up food tasted the best. Potatoes left over from lunch were eaten at night as fried potatoes. On Friday we would eat either fish or a vegetarian dish, according to the Catholic tradition, and on Saturdays we would have *Eintopf*, a soup with ham or sausages and some bread. This custom was probably influenced by the fact that our maid, Else, had Saturdays off. My mother had an occasional glass of wine with dinner, but my father never drank alcohol. Interestingly the identical pattern existed in Linda's family.

On some evenings, as a family, we would play card and table

games. Sometimes we also played ping-pong on the dining room table. My parents would go regularly to the opera, orchestra and theaters. I would go to musicals (operettas) and, with free tickets from our music teacher, to the Sing-Akademie for piano recitals.

On weekends our family went for long walks either in the east (Gruenau, Mueggel See, and Treptow) or in the west (Grunewald, Wannsee, Potsdam). We took the subway or the elevated train to these destinations. We usually would leave after lunch, and then we would have coffee or apple juice and cake at an open-air restaurant. At that time many families would bring their own coffee beans and were allowed to make their own coffee. These restaurants had big signs that said, *Hier koennen Familien Kaffe kochen* (here, families are allowed to brew their own coffee).

My mother was always there for me, and later, for Gisela and my brother, Lothar. Since my father was not a disciplinarian, my mother also had to take over this role, but only very lightly. Mutti was also the person who helped us with most of our homework.

We also visited the *Spreewald* a few times by train, a site that Linda and I later revisited on our trips to Berlin. The Spreewald consists of an area of canals and swamps through which the river Spree flows, and all transportation between houses in the Spreewald occurs by boat.

My father liked to walk, and to walk so fast that my mother had difficulties keeping up. He walked several miles every day, even after retirement. He frequently would also walk to work through the *Lauben Kolonien,* an area full of little garden plots tended by apartment dwellers. Areas like this usually included a *Laube,* a one-room wooden building, a water supply, and I think some kind of a bathroom, but certainly no sewer.

I loved most things about my childhood, but one of the things

I didn't like was my father's persistence to correct my walking and breathing when we went for walks. My father always reminded me to walk upright. "Bru-bru" and "Mu-mu" he would repeat, meaning "chest up" and "breathe through your nose, not your mouth." Vati would also constantly say, "tip, tip," which meant, "do not fall over your feet."

Vati could be quite stubborn. He also bought lots of medical books. From these, he learned about popular medicine; he was particularly dedicated to "deep breathing," "counting to thirty before exhaling," "walking fast" and "chewing each bite thirty times when you eat." Apparently, a professor had written a little book stating that deep breathing was good for the heart. At that time, not many believed him. Now I know that Vati was right. He didn't run in shorts, but his fast walk was almost like a run. You might call him one of the earliest joggers.

At regular times in the winter, we had to sit for a few minutes in front of an ultraviolet lamp to absorb the vitamin D we were missing.

Lembke chocolate factory, where my father worked, sent their chocolates all over Germany. For my father everything but Berlin was "the Province." Towns like Munich and Frankfurt, which after the war became well known, before the war were merely "the Province." This is quite similar to the relationship of Paris to all of France.

Vati liked to paint, mostly watercolors, and he always painted while we were on vacation. Many of his paintings are hanging in my home and the homes of my children. Another of his hobbies was writing poetry and plays. None of them were ever published, with the exception of one small poetry book that Vati self-published. He was religious, in the Lutheran way, and all his poems dealt with

God, duty, family, and love of God. "Love your neighbor as you love yourself," many of his poems proclaimed. Although they are difficult to translate, as they were written in German and in a certain style, here I have attempted to translate one small poem by my father:

Love and Sacrifice

When we are happy and content it is easy to love,
And also easy to be a friend.
No sacrifice is demanded.
There is only sun and blue sky.

Real love shows itself in days,
When life demands sacrifices, when there is pain.
Real love will continue to be present,
Coping with sacrifices quietly and lovingly.

I still have copies of most of his plays and poems and hope that my sons will cherish them, just as I did, even if they are written in German.

My father also carried out an extensive correspondence with the Catholic and Lutheran churches, urging them to unite into one Christian church. He was unsuccessful in this effort. But Vati was an optimist and always positive.

I still can picture Vati walking back and forth in the living room, thinking. And when he had an idea he would sit at his desk and write his thoughts down, either in shorthand or on a typewriter. Mutti read nearly everything he wrote. She had an even more important role whenever Vati smoked a cigar. When he had to go to the bathroom he asked Mutti to continue smoking it so it would not extinguish. When I was a teenager, he gave me his old World War I pipe, which I was allowed only occasionally to smoke.

I was almost eight years old when my sister, Gisela, was born in 1932. My brother, Lothar, was born in 1938. Mutti went to a private clinic for about ten days, and Vati took me to Sande when Gisela was born, and later took Gisela and me somewhere else on vacation when Lothar was born. My father was never at Mutti's bedside when the children were born. My parents felt my father had to be with the other children.

Our new school year always started after two weeks of Easter vacation, comparable to our "Spring Break" vacation in America. During the six weeks of summer vacation our family always spent a few weeks either at the Baltic, primarily on the island of Ruegen, in the village of Goehren, or in the lower German mountains such as the Harz or the Thueringer Wald. At the Baltic, the forest came all the way to the dunes, and we often went into the woods to pick wild blueberries.

In October we then had about ten days *Kartoffel* (potato) vacation. This started years ago to allow the students to work on the farms to help in the potato harvest.

The next vacations came at Christmas time. We had two to three weeks off, beginning before Christmas and lasting until a few days after January 6, *Heilige 3 Koenige* (holy three kings holiday). On December 6, we celebrated St. Nicholas Day, and without fail St. Nicholas brought us a large plate full of cookies, candies, and also healthy food, such as oranges and apples, and a small gift, like a book, for example. The Christmas tree usually was set up on Christmas Eve, and the exchange of gifts was held that evening. We were told as children that the Christ child brought the gifts, with the help of the *Weihnachtsmann* (Santa Claus). The gifts usually appeared while we were at church. In our house we also had the custom to have the advent wreath, with four red candles for the four Sundays before Christmas, on the table; the candles were lighted each Sunday. Candles were red for the four weeks before Christmas and white at Christmas.

The Escalating War

Like everyone else, when I turned ten years old, I joined the Jungvolk, the forerunner of the Hitler Youth, which children usually had to enter at age fourteen. We had classes, walks, games in the woods, campfires and so on. In many ways it must have been like the present-day Boy Scouts. We learned the same outdoor stuff and had similar experiences. When the Jungvolk had something planned on Sundays, I always went to church to the seven o'clock mass. I even went with the Jungvolk to a two-week camp at the Baltic, but soon after I got there I felt homesick. I didn't enjoy the lessons or the activities, and it ended up being the worst experience of my young life. This is probably one of the reasons why I didn't push my own children to go away to summer camp. At age fourteen, when I was supposed to join the Hitler Youth, I was able to get out of it. My parents supported me in that. I had too much schoolwork to do and therefore had no time to join.

I do remember, however, in 1939 when Hitler started World War II by marching into Poland. We were all called into the auditorium of our school and told about this event. The news was met with complete silence. No one showed excitement or applauded. There was only a long silence before we were released to return to our classrooms.

In the winter of 1941, Germany was short on heating material, such as coal, and in the winter the school was only open for a few hours a day. We wore our coats, and classes lasted only fifteen minutes. During that winter I spent several months in Thueringen, helping to oversee elementary students who were evacuated from Berlin because of the frequent air raids. Thueringen's climate is similar to Vermont, and so I always made sure I had my skis with me. I learned later that from 1943 to 1945, my school was closed in Berlin and all children were moved to Silesia in the East, away from the air raids. My sister Gisela's school was also moved to the East, but Gisela stayed in Berlin, and my mother homeschooled her for almost two years. Gisela was twelve years old when the Russians occupied Berlin. My brother Lothar was only seven.

If I remember correctly, the first night that air raids reached Berlin was in late 1940. And by 1941, many children were being sent into the countryside for months at a time to escape the frequent nighttime bombings by the British. The Americans had not yet entered the war, and even after they did it took them some time before they started their daytime bombings. At home, our cellars became air-raid shelters, and this is where we ran from the apartment whenever the air-raid sirens blared. My parents were bombed out in early 1945, and the only things they saved were a few pieces of good china, paintings, and some photos that my parents had kept in the air-raid shelter.

Mutti also managed to save the letters I had sent from my POW camps in America. I later found out that Nana Bee had saved all letters that Linda and I mailed to her during our honeymoon trip through Europe. To my surprise, I discovered that I wrote many more letters than my wife, Linda. And Linda had not only saved my letters written during our courtship, but also all letters she received from Alyssa and Heidi (our daughters-in-law), many written long before either Mike or Steve were married.

Handwritten letters are a lost art these days, replaced by e-mail and other kinds of electronic communication. But I think they're a wonderful way to communicate important, lasting messages—especially to parents. Mothers love to receive and read letters from their children. And if they're like Linda's mother and my mother, they'll hang onto them. Handwritten letters are a gift that keeps giving. They were a treasure when first sent and received, and again when I rediscovered them.

I remember during the war when we collected recyclables like toothpaste tubes and other items in order to help with the war effort. I'm certain we were already suffering from the scarcity of resources even before the war started, since the Nazis had put everything into arms build-up. My ski equipment was also collected for the war in Russia. I started to wear Vati's shirts and suits. During all this time, I was always astounded how many people were openly against the Nazis. As I mentioned earlier, my piano teacher, Mr. Isleib, used up most of the practice time with his students to talk about the terrible Nazis. He liked to remind us that Field Marshall Herman Goering had said that he would change his name to Meyer, a very common name in Germany, if allied planes would ever reach Berlin.

English bombers only came at night, but after the United States entered the war, in late 1941, their bombers mostly attacked during the day. The rail freight yards near our apartment were frequently attacked by the Allied flyers. Yet, no matter how many bombers came, all public transportation continued to run. Even when damaged by bombs, swift repairs assured transportation would be functioning within a very short period of time. This was the case, I was told, even toward the end of the war when much more damage was caused by the bombings. I wonder how a large city in America would have reacted to such continuous bombing.

As the war extended into the fall of 1941, my father sat me down and said, "Karl-Heinz, we have to talk about the war." I was always called "Karl-Heinz" in Germany, even though my baptized name was only Karl. The story is that my mother's father's name was Heinrich, and my father hated that name and didn't want it on the birth certificate. However, he made a compromise with my mother and agreed to call me Karl-Heinz instead of Karl. My school friends, however, always called me Kalle. And once I joined the army, I was always Karl only.

My father continued, "Karl-Heinz, Germany will lose the war. By whom would you rather be captured during, or at the end of, the war, the Russians, or the British in Africa?" There was no question that the British were the only choice. "Well, if you want to become a prisoner of war of the British, you have to make sure you can fight the war in Africa under Rommel. In order to achieve this goal, you have to follow a rather circuitous route.

"First, do not wait until you are drafted. Instead, you have to volunteer for the army. This will allow you to select the type of service you want to get into. Second, volunteer to become an officer, which will guarantee you more time training in Germany, and also will allow you to select the theater of operation in which you want to fight."

By sheer luck an old friend of my mother from high school was a lieutenant colonel in the Signal Corps in Potsdam, near Berlin, where all basic training for the Berlin area took place. He was in charge of the basic training for the Signal Corps. My mother contacted him, and he advised her that I should apply to his unit for training, and he would help me select either the wireless or the telephone unit.

And thus, after I completed high school with my Abitur in March 1942, I joined the Army Signal Corp and went to Potsdam for boot camp. All volunteers lined up on the parade grounds, and a sergeant divided us into two groups, wireless or telephone. I was placed into the wireless group, but I preferred the other. So, on the pretense of having to use the bathroom, I went to the colonel's office and requested to be assigned to the telephone part of the Signal Corps. He arranged it, and I started my three months of basic training in my preferred subunit of the Signal Corps.

And so, at the young age of 17, I learned these important lessons: never give up, and go for what you want.

The first day in the army, I learned that the army hated the Nazis. The sergeant in charge inquired, "Who here had a leadership role in the Hitler Youth?" Several recruits raised their hands. He told them, "Run twenty times around the whole column. This shows you how we like your organization."

After twelve weeks of basic training, I was moved to the officers' training school, also in Potsdam. This training lasted for six months. During that time all of the men in our unit contracted scarlet fever, and we were quarantined for three weeks in barracks right on a big lake.

During my officer training, I learned to drive big trucks, buses, regular cars, and motorbikes. After the war, the army driver's license helped me get a German license to drive whatever was allowed on the road. I was fortunate to spend weekends during this six-month training period at home with my parents. And then, before being shipped to Africa, I used my vacation days to visit Greifswald, my father's relatives, and later also Willich, my mother's relatives.

Before I could go to officers' candidate school, I had to have at least three months frontline experience.

I expected to have that soon enough. But sometimes, life has other plans.

2

Prisoner of War (POW) in America

I was promoted to Private First Class (Pfc) and Reserve Officer Bewerber (ROB) candidate on December 15, 1942, after completing and passing the officers' candidate-training course.

In the middle of January 1943, I received my travel papers for Africa, specifically for Signal Corps 475, the Signal Corp of the Africa Corps under the command of Field Marshall Rommel. Another officer candidate and I traveled by express train from Berlin to Naples around the middle of February, changing in Rome for the Naples train. We traveled second class. It was comfortable and exciting, having window seats the whole time. We wore our new Africa Corps uniforms and were proud to join such an elite army group. I was just eighteen.

In Naples we reported to one of the best hotels on the promenade overlooking the harbor. It was requisitioned by the German Army as a holding station for soldiers who needed transport to Africa. We stayed in Naples for a couple of weeks (I didn't step on

African soil until March 11). Our days were free, and we explored
Naples, including the church with the Madonna picture whose
eyes always follow you; and old Naples with the laundry hanging
across narrow streets, where eight-year-old boys were pimping their
twelve-year-old, or younger, sisters. There was nearly no war damage, and stores in Italy were still full of goods one could no longer
buy in Germany. I bought silk stockings, gloves, and all kinds of
other things for my mother and mailed them to Berlin. And, indeed, they did arrive. The black market was very active in Naples,
but I do not remember much about it.

Suddenly our papers for Africa arrived. We were herded into a
Junkers 52, the three-engine workhorse of the Luftwaffe transport
system. I sat at a window next to a machine gun and was instructed
to use it properly when attacked by British planes. Luckily no one
attacked us, and after a short flight we arrived in Tunis, the capital of
Tunisia. We were on our own, with marching papers in our hands,
and we hitchhiked for about a week until we reached the unit to
which we were assigned. When I reached the front lines, the Africa
Corps already had retreated from El Alamein to far beyond Tobruk.
The British Air Force clearly controlled the sky by the time I arrived
in North Africa. So the whole time I was in Africa, I was basically
on retreat from the British Eighth Army, headed by Montgomery.
North Africa, and particularly Tunisia, was a beautiful and exciting
country—strange, yet compelling. (The time in Africa must have
impressed me, as I initially remembered being in Africa much longer, at least four months.) The German Army always dealt fairly
with the local Arabs in the area. We could not simply take eggs or
chickens or other food away from them, we had to pay for everything. I was assigned to a group whose job it was to string telephone
wires and to repair them.

We were three men, a sergeant and two soldiers, and we traveled in a big SUV. My primary job was to string telephone lines from the front lines to headquarters. Since British airplanes strafed the German lines, we usually dug foxholes in which to sleep at night. In the desert, the days were so hot we fried eggs on the cars' hoods. The nights, however, were bitter cold. We slept in sweaters, winter coats, and under blankets. Our men's room was the desert. We dug a hole in the ground and that was our toilet.

We were stationed opposite the British, but in the aftermath of the battle of the Kasserine Pass, we were also thrown into the battle. Here I could observe first-hand the tremendous power of the 88 mm anti-aircraft gun, which could level and destroy any tank.

The most loved song at the time, by both the Germans and the British, was "Lili Marlene," which was played on both German and British Army radio stations. This was a song about a young soldier going to war, saying goodbye to his girlfriend. Their last embrace was under the street light in front of the soldiers' barracks. He was leaving for the war, perhaps not to come back, but his girl would wait under the street light in front of the barracks.

Lili Marlene

Underneath the lantern,
By the barrack gate,
Darling I remember
The way you used to wait.
'Twas there that you whispered tenderly
That you loved me,
You'd always be,
My Lili of the Lamplight,
My own Lili Marlene

Time would come for roll call,
Time for us to part,
Darling I'd caress you
And press you to my heart,
And there 'neath that far-off lantern light,
I'd hold you tight,
We'd kiss good night,
My Lili of the Lamplight,
My own Lili Marlene[1]

I still listen to it sometimes, as I have it on a CD in my car.

We had a chance to visit old cities such as Sfax and Kairuan, including the holy temples, and we had to behave well and act honorably.

The desert impressed me, though it was little more than sand hills and wadis, dried out rivers that flowed only a short time during the year during the rainy season. I did not experience rain. We ate stale rye bread and for hot meals, mutton with rice. We also had to take salt pills daily because of the heat.

My *Soldbuch*, a personal record every German soldier carried with him, had recorded such items as home address, army unit, rank, promotions, vacations, weapons and clothing issued. I still find it interesting to note what is listed there. I originally had a rifle, and when I entered officers training, I received a pistol. I also had a gas mask. I received the following items for my time in Africa: a hat (similar to a baseball cap); two jackets; two pairs of pants, one with normal legs and one to wear with our boots; a pair of short pants; three underwear shorts; one olive warm coat; three shirts with collars; three undershirts; one nightgown; one scarf to protect the neck from the sun; one tie; one woolen sweater; three blankets; four pair of socks; two pair of warm socks; one shirt (not further described); one set of suspenders; one backpack; one mosquito net; one gnat scarf; one sleeping bag; and several utensils, such as a water flask, eating utensils, and a belt. We also received one bed sheet, three hankies, one towel, one work cloth outfit, equipment to set up a tent, and one signal whistle. I was vaccinated for small pox, cholera, and typhus/paratyphus, and my height was recorded as 180 cm (5'11").

The war in Africa ended May 12, 1943. General Oberst von Arnim, a four star general, served as the Africa Corps commander after Rommel went home for sick leave. It was von Arnim who signed the unconditional surrender, and it happened just a few months after Stalingrad surrendered to the Russians. The British Eighth Army captured me, but we were at once turned over to the Americans. We were happy that the war was over for us. At the same time, we were scared and worried about the future and what would happen to us. There was a lot of uncertainty.

The air was full of rumors. We were herded into large open spaces surrounded by barbed wire, receiving tents as shelters only much later. Roll calls, several times daily, and strip searches, almost daily, seemed to occupy us. The rest of the day we just sat around and waited—for what we did not yet know.

A day after the war in Africa was over, and before enlisted men and officers were separated, a German general promoted me to "corporal and officers candidate of the reserve" and had my captain enter this promotion into my soldier's book. At that time I was also awarded the Italian Memorial Medal and the Africa Armband. One or two months later I would have returned to Germany to complete the last step of my officer training. But this did not happen.

Discovering America

One of my first impressions of the Americans was that they had more air-conditioned food trucks than tanks. But it was another impression that really captured my attention. Once among the Americans, we received the first good meal since entering North Africa. We received ice-cold potato salad, the best hot dogs I have ever eaten, and vanilla ice cream! If I would not have known it before, I certainly knew then that the United States would win the war.

Early captivity was a confusing, stressful time, defined perhaps most notably by rumors and hearsay. We were kept in large holding areas surrounded by barbed wire. We had frequent roll calls, were constantly checked for hidden weapons, and the American soldiers wondered aloud why we had no horns (as the "Huns" had been described in American newspapers). The Africa Corps was an elite unit similar to elite units in the American Army, and in contrast to what many believed, we never were Nazis; we were German soldiers belonging to the elite Africa Corps.

Life as a prisoner of war was marked by an unsettling boredom. We had nothing to do but stand or sit around and eat. We had many guards, though I didn't understand this since we were all happy that the war was over for us. After a time, we were moved by truck through Tunisia and ended up in a camp that I will never forget. We were stripped naked, our belongings were searched, and all valuables confiscated. I had a few cuff links and a pocket watch from my grandfather, protected against the desert sands by a tight casing. We received receipts for our belongings, but never expected to see anything again. I was allowed to keep my high school English book and my English dictionary—books my father made me take with me to Africa. These books became invaluable to me. Early on in my captivity, I spent all my free time trying to improve my English. I studied the books and spoke as often as I could with our guards. Since not many German soldiers spoke English, I saw a golden future, namely to become an interpreter, and with this I would be able to more easily assume leadership positions in the camp.

We were moved by freight train through an area full of vineyards and fruit farms to the Tunisian coast at Bone, where we embarked on a troop transport ship that took us to Oran, Morocco. From there we were shipped by truck to a large tent camp, a holding camp, until transportation to America could be arranged. Now, we finally knew that we would head for American soil soon.

A few weeks later (by now it was mid-June 1943) we were transported again to the harbor of Oran, where we were loaded on liberty ships full of German prisoners in their holds sailing to America. We slept on blankets on the floor in the cargo holds. During daytime we were permitted on deck, which allowed us to improve on our African tans. After we crossed the strait of Gibraltar, a ship convoy was established with destroyers and a cruiser for protection. Suddenly, German submarines attacked us, and for the first time, I prayed for the Americans and not the Germans.

The trip took about three weeks and was otherwise uneventful. We had the best weather. The food was not that great, as there was no kitchen on the ship other than for the crew, since these ships were actually ammunition and freight ships, not transport ships. But we received ample supplies of cold, American Army K-rations.

After our arrival in Newport News, Virginia, in the summer of 1943, we swiftly disembarked, went through a de-licing station, were stripped and sprayed with DDT, then were registered and received our POW number (8WG-22939). I was one of the first soldiers from Africa who arrived in America. After being fed, we entered elegant Pullman cars for our three-day train trip to Camp Swift, Texas. In each car was a US soldier with a gun, and we had to ask permission to go to the bathroom or even just to move around. Otherwise it was a comfortable trip in plush seats. We had plenty to eat and to drink.

Camp Swift

I had come down with hepatitis on the trip, and so as soon as we got to Camp Swift, I was sent to the hospital. My hepatitis was treated with rest and with a high-carbohydrate diet. Thanks to my father's wisdom in making me bring my English books, I soon became the hospital interpreter. I had this job for a year, until we were transferred to Camp Somerset in Maryland to help in the harvest and in canning factories.

In the hospital I met Johann Kleist, a POW my age who also had come from Africa, and with whom I still have contact. In fact, several decades later, Johann and his wife came to the wedding of my son, Mike, and his wife, Alyssa.

At Camp Swift I worked hard to replace my book-learned English with American idioms and words. Once I asked our nurse whether she had taken a *douche,* which I quickly learned in English meant something quite different from a *shower.* We all laughed. While an interpreter in the Camp Swift hospital, a young army nurse seduced me. Thus, I was initiated into adult life around the time I turned nineteen.

After I'd been at Camp Swift for about three months, to my great surprise, all of my private belongings that had been taken away in Africa, arrived. When this happened, I was once again convinced that America would win the war. Surely this was the most honest and efficient country in the world. This was probably the first time that I thought about returning to America after the war.

Most Sundays we went to church, and I still have the small pocket Bible that the Catholic army chaplain gave me as a gift soon after my arrival in Camp Swift. In the spring of 1944, I experienced a severe acne attack. I was treated by an American dermatologist; I received ultraviolet rays as treatment and medication, just like any American soldier would have been treated.

Camp Swift consisted of rows of barracks and open spaces, surrounded by wire fences and guard towers. There were special barracks for the mess hall, bathrooms, latrines, library, post-exchange (PX), laundry, and entertainment. Germans usually ran all of the POW camps under the direction of American guards. Many of the German camp chiefs were sergeants, frequently Nazis, and luckily as an interpreter, I was beyond their reach. Every morning and every evening we had roll calls, as if we planned to escape. However, I was fortunate to have many opportunities to leave the camp to meet with civilians. We were allowed to write and receive weekly letters, but only until the end of the war in Europe. For our work we received seventy-five cents a day, which we could spend at the PX.

As you may expect, sex was a big topic of discussion for young men in captivity. Many of the stories told, I am sure, were fiction rather than truth. The story of one man sticks particularly in my mind. I believe it impressed me at that time. He was recently married when a girlfriend of his wife visited them. Since they had only one bedroom, the wife and girlfriend suggested that they all sleep in the bed together. While the wife's friend was still awake, he and his wife had wild sex. This excited the friend so much that, once the wife was asleep, she also wanted sex. And so, in the same bed, the soldier had his second round of sex. Such boasts of sexual prowess were as common as roll calls.

The atmosphere in the camps wasn't all fun and games, though. After the invasions of Sicily and Italy, some hardcore Nazis were captured and sent to American POW camps, which made life miserable for many. Our enemies were never the Americans, but the small groups of German Nazis.

I remember in particular when a Nazi subgroup became quite powerful in Camp Swift. This prompted the army to break the prisoners up, shipping some to other camps. It was also around this time that orders came from above that POWs should work not only for the army, but for private employers, as America had lost many laborers to the war effort.

Camp Somerset

When I was shipped to Camp Somerset in June 1944, my friend Johann, who worked in the mess hall at Camp Swift, was also transferred. In Maryland, most prisoners worked in chicken and canning factories or in the fields. Lots of interesting stories came back to camp with the workers. I remember one from workers in the chicken factory. Since the production line in chicken factories ran very fast, occasionally a chicken would be hung up without first being killed, or the head would be cut off, but the headless body was left flying around the factory, blood spilling on the prisoners.

The day we arrived, the new commander asked whether any of us had worked in a ration detail before. I raised my hand and said, "I have." I hadn't, but this seemed like a harmless enough lie. From that moment on I became the chief of the ration detail, providing all food supplies for the German and American mess halls. I drove my own half-ton truck and worked closely with two GIs supplying both kitchens. We ordered our bread from a local bakery and would pick up most of the other food in Fort Meade on the Chesapeake Bay. I was allowed to spend some evenings outside the camp with my American partners. I visited some bars, bought shoes and other clothing. I also joined my American friends in a little black market activity.

We had a wonderful relationship with our guards. I still have photos from a show that some prisoners gave for the other prisoners and the American guards. The American Camp Commander was great. Our camp security was relaxed. We read *The New York Times*; listened to the radio; and played ping-pong, chess, and soccer. We were not restricted at all. We were treated just like our American guards. In the PX we could buy cigarettes, chocolate, tobacco, beer, Coke, and other items in whatever quantities we wanted. This was also true for soap, shaving material, and toilet articles.

An American radio commentator, Walter Winchell, complained that the German prisoners were "swimming in butter" while butter was being rationed for the civilians. Yet even his tirade against the "babying of the prisoners" did not change anything. Fraternization between guards and prisoners continued. We were all soldiers, not politicians. None of us soldiers started the war. Camaraderie just developed. We all wanted the war to end so that we could go home and get on with our lives.

Later, when I was at Huntsville, Texas, working as the leader and interpreter of a work detail, our American guards who accompanied us to our outside work details would even lend me a gun to protect the detail while they slept. I was allowed to shoot armadillos and other animals, but had to promise to clean the gun. I always did.

A lot of my memories from Camp Somerset come from letters I

wrote to my parents (which my mother thankfully saved). In a letter to my parents, dated August 9, 1944, I said, "English perfect." In a letter dated August 28, I wrote, "Do not worry about me, 'weeds' do not disappear." It's important to note that all my letters were rather artificial, since they were censored before being sent and we weren't allowed to say much. It usually took about two months for mail between American camps and Berlin. It was transported back and forth by the Swiss Red Cross.

In a letter dated October 14, I complained that it was getting cold, and that we had to wear our woolen pants and our wind jackets. In November I wrote about a big party in the camp, complete with Coke, beer, coffee, cake, a band, and plenty of ice cream.

In a letter sent in November I wrote, "Johann and I are the ping-pong champions of our camp." In my last letter from Somerset I wrote, "I am sitting in an easy chair in the library, listening to radio from the Metropolitan Opera, and reading *The New York Times*." In the afternoon we had soccer matches. The supper included pumpernickel that I arranged through my ration detail.

While Johann stayed in Somerset until the end of the war, I was transferred in December 1944 to Camp Huntsville, Texas, which was established as a non-commissioned officer's camp. I wrote this in my first letter from Camp Huntsville: "No work, boring, nothing to do."

Camp Huntsville and Camp China

It was January 1945 that I reported to my mother that I'd just won a chess tournament. We played lots of chess in camp; we also played various card games, poker and volleyball. In Huntsville, cigarettes started to be rationed to eighty per week. Food quality had decreased a bit, too, but it was still much better than I could have hoped for. For a few months after the war ended, food and other supplies were rationed, but the restrictions were eventually relaxed before the end of the year.

One of the things I remember best about my Camp Huntsville experience was our weekly movie. I was appointed movie interpreter. American movies had to be screened by the German leadership and German movies by the American leadership. As the chief interpreter I also had to teach the other, lower-level interpreters so they could interpret US movies to the German prisoners in real time while the movie was playing.

In March 1945, I was moved to a branch camp, Camp China, Texas, run by my friend, Captain Smith, where I worked in one of the largest US nurseries and did some interpreting for him. We shipped plant material all over the United States. I drove a large American car and spent all my time interpreting and supervising. For Easter we sent gardenias or camellias, I do not remember which, to New York.

April was frighteningly hot. It was also a rather eventful month, as we spent a week fighting river flooding in Beaumont, Texas, by filling and placing sandbags. It was hard work, but also exciting.

Captain Smith went on vacation in May and gave me time off, as I had worked so well. His temporary replacement did not like this arrangement and assigned me as a laborer to a lumber detail, cutting pine trees to be shipped to paper mills. I learned to cut trees with handsaws worked by two men, and also to use an axe to make the tree fall in the direction we wanted it to fall. Our detail had to produce two and a half cords per day. I learned a lot and became an accomplished lumberjack.

At the water barrel that held the ice water we drank to hydrate, I experienced an incident that I will never forget. We worked together with black laborers. There was a really big and strong black man who was always helpful to us, and we liked him. So, on one very hot day we were both taking a much-needed rest. I offered him the ladle to drink some ice water. The guard came swiftly and took the ladle away from the black worker. The POWs could drink from the same ladle as the guards, but he would not allow a black man to drink from the same ladle as the whites. They had their own barrel—full of lukewarm water. This was a shock to me, and it was the first time I became aware of the severity of the race problems in America.

In Camp China, we slept in tents on top of a wooden contraption waist high on all sides of the tent and with a wooden floor. Our beds had netting to keep the mosquitoes away. After fourteen days Captain Smith returned from his vacation and he took me at once out of the lumber detail. I became the interpreter of a large wood-cutting detail and did not have to work hard labor anymore. Instead, I took care of the records and the books.

Once the war ended in Europe, we were required to see movies about the KZ, or concentration camps. They were horrible. We never knew anything about the KZ camps while in Germany or Africa. They also shipped guards to us who had been prisoners of war in Germany, hoping that fraternization would now stop. But these former US prisoners in Germany were very nice to us and said they were treated as well in Germany as the German soldiers were treated in Germany, which was rather poorly, indeed. I wrote home that work was ten hours a day, and if one did not fulfill his quota, he would not get breakfast. I personally don't remember such strict treatment by American authorities, but then, my detail always fulfilled its quota.

From September to November I was appointed interpreter and

leader of a detail working for the largest rice farmer in the area. The farmer had heard about me and requested me from Captain Smith. He was one of the richest farmers and had several ranches in other states, and also owned many oil wells. During the summer and fall of 1945, many prisoners, particularly those working cutting trees, lost weight because they had very little to eat. But the rice farmers fed us lunch and allowed us to bring rice back into the camps to the mess hall. Once November came, all prisoners were fed well again.

The rice detail consisted of fifteen POWs and twenty-five blacks. I rode a horse and sometimes drove in a car, either alone or with the farmer's ten-year-old son. I supervised the harvest. His wife invited me home to her house for tea. It was a wonderful experience.

In addition to the rice, the farmer also often gave us beer and wine. He took me to bars in town. And the farmer cooked warm lunches for us. Since tobacco was scarce at that time, the farmer and the blacks shared their tobacco and cigarettes with us. When the harvest was over, the farmer arranged a celebration with liquor and food and cigarettes. The whole detail got drunk. He gave me a bottle of a very rare Scottish whiskey.

Rumors had been swirling in camp ever since the end of the war. Some American papers talked about sending us as slaves to France and England. These rumors prompted me to seek out more information as soon as I heard about the Fort Eustis anti-Nazi course for a rather select group of POWs. And once I learned about it, I knew I would have to attend this course. In fact, I later learned that my friend Johann was sent from America for another year of captivity to England to work on the farms. He did not go to Fort Eustis.

When Camp China was closed, we did not return to Huntsville, since Huntsville also was being closed, but were assigned to Camp Polk, Louisiana. Here, food and supplies were again bountiful. We received excellent treatment. The only problems we had there were with the German camp leadership. Simply stated: dumb sergeants.

Captain Smith took me along as his interpreter. He said to me, "Karl, we have to find some anti-Nazis, can you think of some?" I responded, "Yes, one, me." I helped him to select prisoners for the democratic training course in Fort Eustis, Virginia, and put myself at the top of the list, to which the captain agreed. Selection was based on lack of party membership, behavior as a POW, education, participation in religious activities, and knowledge of English. A rather intensive and complex questionnaire had to be completed which was evaluated at Fort Eustis long before we arrived. Many prisoners proposed for the course were rejected, either before even arriving in Fort Eustis or after their arrival, before the course started.

Fort Eustis and Home

It was now the end of 1945. There was nothing to do but wait to go to Fort Eustis and then, home. Over the next three months, more than twenty thousand POWs went through the six day Fort Eustis course. Upon completion, we received a certificate stating that we had passed the Fort Eustis course—that we were good Germans—and were considered to be ready to help the occupying authorities in the rebuilding of Germany.

The course was impressive. It wasn't just propaganda. We saw films of the Holocaust, but also learned the good and bad things about America. The approach was honest, sincere, and had a great educational impact on me. We concluded the week with a celebration and received a Fort Eustis certificate, which I have lost. I had it in Germany, but cannot find it anymore.

Participation in the course guaranteed I could go home to Germany. Others either had to work in America until July, or were sent to work in England or France.

The program at Fort Eustis focused on twelve topics:

1. The democratic way of life
2. The Constitution of the United States
3. Political parties, election, and parliamentary procedures
4. Education in the United States
5. American family life
6. The American economic scene
7. American military government
8. Democratic traditions in Germany
9. Why the Weimar Republic failed-Part I
10. Why the Weimar Republic failed-Part II
11. The world of today and Germany
12. New democratic trends in the world today[2]

We received a barrack bag, several woolen blankets, a first-aid kit, eating utensils, and so on. But we had to leave much behind, such as radios, field glasses, knives, and cigarette lighters. We were now waiting for transport ships to become available. These ships arrived in the US filled with American troops returning home from Europe, and it returned to Europe filled with German POWs.

From Ft. Eustis, we were transferred via two camps, Camp Patrick Henry and Fort Shanks, both in New York State, to our transfer ship for Europe, waiting for us in New York. I was appointed the leader of one, with 1,500 prisoners being shipped home to Europe via our transport ship. This happened, thanks to an American captain whom I knew quite well. I lived on the ship in a private room in the infirmary. I was registered in Berlin as a medical student, which now made me the "young doctor." We had great food and enjoyed many movies in the movie theater for the Americans. The trip took nine days. I learned from POWs on other transport ships that our ship had much better meals than other ships that left at the same time.

After we arrived in France, we were transported by trucks to Camp Bolbec, forty miles from Le Havre. From Le Havre I had smuggled a letter to my parents with an American friend, who mailed it for me in Bremen. While many prisoners were sent to France for work in the mines or on the farms, and others were directly sent from America to England for farm work, the Fort Eustis prisoners were accompanied by American officers to make sure that the French or the British would not divert us for further work in their countries.

After arrival at Bolbec we were supposed to leave within a day or two for Bad Aibling, Bavaria, which was the American camp from which all US prisoners were discharged. But there were no trains available, so we just laid around in camp for two weeks. We lived in tents on straw, but without beds. When it rained, and it rained a lot—torrential rain—we got soaked from the wet floor. It was a tough time. After several days, three transport chiefs (including me), each representing about 1,200 prisoners from Fort Eustis, were able to persuade the American camp administration to provide us with beds. This had never happened before. But several days after we got the beds, we suddenly had to prepare for the transport to Germany.

Our American captain, who had accompanied us from Fort Eustis, told us that beginning the next day one train would leave per day. Since trains could handle more men than our 1,200 transport group, our old groups were re-divided. I was scheduled for the second trip. When we marched to our transport train consisting of freight cars, my captain, the transport officer, saw me, called me out of the ranks, and asked me to climb into his jeep. I joined him, another American officer, two German officers, and several sick prisoners in a special railroad car. The food aboard the train was excellent. It took two-and-a-half days to travel to Bad Aibling. After six days there, we were discharged by the Americans.

POWs had to choose into which of the three Western Zones (American, British, or French) they wanted to be discharged, as it was impossible to be discharged to Berlin and the Russian Zone (Eastern). I selected the British Zone where my mother's relatives lived. On May 3, those who planned to settle in the British Zone traveled there by transport train to be discharged by the British in a few days. Since we were already discharged, we were simply awaiting a stamp on our papers, and then, our freedom. However, as soon as we arrived at the British prisoner discharge camp Munsterlager, we were stripped down and examined like real prisoners. The British took much of our savings away, claiming it would go to the United Nations Relief and Rehabilitation Administration (UNRA). People ill or unable to work were discharged in a few days. The healthy ones were told they would be shipped to England for farm work. Fort Eustis meant nothing to the British Army personnel and their German help running the POW discharge camp. When German physicians examined us for fitness to work in England, I played it safe. I pointed to my scar from the motorbike accident many years ago, said that I had always headaches and dizziness, and that I was a medical student. He was sympathetic and declared me "unfit" for work. I still have my discharge papers.

Since all Eustis graduates were supposed to have been discharged right away, we sneaked two prisoners out of the camp and sent them by freight train to Frankfurt to the Americans for help. Two days later a young American lieutenant arrived, raised a stink, and in two days we were all discharged. We even received some of our stuff back that had been taken away from us just a few days earlier. Once again I was reminded that the Americans were clearly in charge of the war. The British had to give in.

A nine-hour trip by train took us to Muenster, the next largest city to our discharge camp. Today, the trip would probably take only two hours. Remember, it was May 1946, and Germany lay in ruins. There we stayed for two days. The German sergeant did not want to let me go to the university, but I went to the British officer, and he gave me a daily pass. I looked around at the university, where I was told that no medical first semester was offered, only science.

I had always wanted to study medicine and was matriculated in Berlin University as a medical student by mail from my POW camp. This did not help me, and it was all the more important for me that I start medical school right away and not lose half a year. I had already lost too much time as it was. I was now almost twenty-two years old.

From Muenster, we travelled by truck to Krefeld. From Krefeld I traveled by streetcar to Willich. Finally, on May 22, I was a free man!

Thinking back on my time in the German Army and my three years as a POW in America, I have mostly good memories. It would be easy to think of these four years as a loss, but instead, I see them as an important part of my life. *This experience allowed me to grow and mature, to become self-reliant, to learn to fight for things I wanted, and not to worry about the things I could not change. When I started medical school at nearly twenty-two years old, I was probably more mature than those who did not have these experiences.* And, of course, I came through the war alive. Indeed, I was a very lucky young man.

I later learned that most of my former classmates were either killed during the war or taken prisoner by the Russians, most of them dying in camps. Listening to my father's advice in early 1942 saved my life and gave me the chance to appreciate and love America.

Back to Germany, Back to School

I arrived in Willich on May 22, 1946, finally a free man. The last mail I had received from my parents when in America was dated February 20, 1945.

I registered in Willich the first day I arrived in order to become a citizen of the town. My aunts were very happy, as the authorities wanted to send them a stranger to use their extra room. For five years Willich was my home. My aunts and uncle took care of me as if I were their son. They spoiled me rotten. I still have some of their antique family furniture from 1750, which I inherited after all three had passed away.

While the British took much away from us, I still was able to save some things. I mailed tobacco, soap, shaving cream, and razor blades to Vati; a toothbrush, toothpaste, and fine soap to Mutti; and chocolates for Lothar and Gisela. For Aunt Kaetchen and Aunt Hanna I had cigarettes and real coffee. I had an American equivalent of $240, for which I received almost one thousand *Reichsmark*.

I had managed to save this amount of money from a daily pay of seventy-five cents.

I couldn't get ration cards for clothing until June. Uncle Richard was still in captivity when I arrived, and I wore one of his suits. My parents were in the Russian sector in Berlin, but I was registered in the British Zone as a refugee from the East. This had some advantages in getting ration coupons for clothing. Uncle Max also gave me a suit of his and a dress shirt. I gave Uncle Max twenty cigarettes for this. Socks and underwear I had already from America, as well as a sweater. I brought along black woolen pants and a wind jacket without POW stamped on them, and a winter coat with the POW stamp. Aunt Kaetchen hoped to get rid of the stamp, but I don't remember whether or not she was successful. I wore the coat anyway.

Willich was a small town of fewer than ten thousand people. It was connected by streetcar to Krefeld, a town of about 175,000. Krefeld was at least 50 percent bombed out, but trains were running. Willich was not bombed out at all. At that time, Willich was surrounded by large farms. Many farmers were friends of my relatives, and I frequently rode my bike to them to pick up milk, butter, and other foods, often bartering for these items. In our townhouse uncle Richard had a drugstore and photo lab, and Aunt Kaetchen had a hardware and china store. Aunt Hanna was office manager of an accounting firm that did taxes for large companies, including Bols in the Netherlands. Therefore, even in 1946 we always had Bols liquor for our own use.

Sunday was always an interesting day in Willich, a primarily Catholic town. While the elderly men and women and the younger women went to church before the Mass began, most younger men met for a beer in the Huette, a small tavern located in the shadow of the church. They waited for the church bell to ring at the end of the sermon, then went to the church for a few minutes, just in time for the offering and communion. Then they all returned to the Huette, having fulfilled their weekly Mass obligation. This was rather typical for a small Catholic town at that time. Church, prayer, and raising children was considered the "woman's job."

Surprisingly, despite all the destruction, trains and streetcars ran at regular schedule, but buses hardly existed, as they needed unavailable gasoline.

The day after arriving in Willich, I traveled by train to Bonn to look at the university, upon recommendation from someone in Willich. I also had to do something for Uncle Max in Bonn, and was home again in the evening for Aunt Hanna's birthday, when I gave her as a gift a carton of American cigarettes. The dean of admissions at Bonn assured me that I could join them for the winter semester, but said he had no opening for the spring semester. Aunt Kaetchen had a friend in Muenster who was a urologist and assistant professor. Uncle Max also had a friend from the army who lived there. I was told I could stay there as needed during the first semester. I now planned to try my luck in Muenster.

So, the next day I decided to go to Muenster, about one hundred kilometers northeast in Westphalia. I was hoping I still might be able to get admitted for the summer semester, even though it had started a month earlier. From Willich, I took the streetcar to Krefeld railway station at six o'clock in the morning. The station was bombed out. From there I took a train to Essen in the Ruhr valley, and then transferred to a train to Muenster. When I arrived in Muenster, there *was* no train station. Just a bunch of train tracks. Everything had been bombed out, but the trains were still running. Nearly 80 percent of Muenster had been destroyed in the war. Only a famous church in the center of town, the Lamberti church, was almost untouched, but the cathedral was heavily damaged. Even the university had been bombed out. The apartment buildings in the outskirts were still standing, and thankfully, the university hospital in the outskirts of Muenster had nearly no damage. In 1946, classes for the whole university were held almost exclusively at the hospital.

Since Muenster was so heavily damaged, many students lived in villages around Muenster and came to classes by train. The students had also created a new walk to the clinics, where all other faculties had their lectures and seminars. This walk was a straight line through town, where buildings formerly stood. It wasn't a real road. It reminded me of the Forum Romanum in Rome, where you walk through 2,000-year-old ruins.

There were a few buildings still standing—a few houses and a couple restaurants—yet most of them were full of bullet holes and bomb damage. I followed the walking pass through the ruins to the building that housed the department of orthopedics. The dean of admissions for the medical school was in that building. After being turned down for the summer semester by the office staff for having applied much too late, I appealed to the dean. He, too, turned me away. And so I found out where the British military government was located and tracked down the British university officer, Mr. Perraudin, in charge of university affairs. My Fort Eustis certificate opened a door to see the British university officer. He told me, "Mr. Rickels, I cannot tell the university authorities what to do, but I can ask them to view your application as if you were one of the earliest ones who had applied." He wrote this recommendation on his official stationery. I still today see it in front of me, "His Majesty's Service" in big block letters at the top. I returned with this letter to the dean of admissions. When he read this letter, he almost stood at attention, and I was admitted that same day. Ah, the power of authority!

Medical School

For the first semester, which lasted from late April to the end of July, classes were held for four days every two weeks. In the spring of 1946, most of the universities were newly reopened after having been closed for several years during the war. Many of the buildings were destroyed by bombs, and so the schools were only open intermittently to accommodate classes as they were able.

I stayed for these four days at uncle Max's friend's home, sleeping on the living room couch and paying him rent of thirty Reichsmark a month. It was about a thirty-minute walk to the hospital. The apartment building where he lived was far from the center of town and therefore survived the bombings unscathed.

Halfway to the hospital was the student cafeteria, where, with ration coupons, we received soup to eat. The German economy was run by ration coupons for almost everything until the summer of 1948. The ration cards allowed a close to starvation diet of 900–1200 calories per day. Black-marketing and bartering helped the many lucky ones to improve on these meager ration cards. Without advance warning, and without telling American and British occupation authorities, the economics minister, Dr. Ehrhardt, cancelled the use of all ration cards and initiated the currency reform overnight. Only a small amount of the old Reichsmark could be converted at the ratio of 10:1 into the new Deutsche Mark. The currency reform became an immediate success and laid the groundwork for the German recovery.

The cafeteria was located on a beautiful lake where, before the war, students used to sail. The first semester I was registered in a PhD program of biological sciences, since medicine was not yet read in the first two semesters. However, since only nonmedical subjects are taught in the first year of medical school, I was sure that my courses would be accepted later, and they were. After the first year of medical school, I passed the Vor-Physikum (zoology, botany, chemistry, and physics). One year later I passed the Physikum (biochemistry, anatomy, physiology, microbiology). Although I don't know how it's done today, at that time in Germany all examinations were given orally. Four students would be given the one-hour exam at the same time by the head professor of a given department. When finally completing the clinical part of medical school, all exams were handled the same way as our Physikum exams.

After the first two years of medical school, we focused the next three years primarily on clinical subjects. Medical school consisted of lectures, patient presentations during lectures, and to a lesser degree, seminars and minimal practical experience such as history-taking, auscultation and percussion, ECG interpretations, ophthalmological evaluation, and so on.

One funny incident sticks in my mind. One of the medical students got so nervous during ophthalmological examination of his patient that he could not see anything. Suddenly he remembered how the retina of the eye looks under the microscope and described this finding to the instructor as if he were seeing it with his ophthalmoscope. Whereupon the instructor responded, "Mr. Colleague, you should have your eyes patented, they are so extremely strong!"

Most clinical experience occurred during semester vacations, where we worked in recognized teaching hospitals. I spent one summer in surgery at the Catholic hospital in Krefeld, and another at the internal medicine department in a new county hospital in Sande, where I also had a room and board for free. I spent my OB-GYN time again in Krefeld.

Between semesters I also worked on my doctoral dissertation in the laboratory of Professor Lintzel in Krefeld. My topic was sulfur-containing amino acids in soybeans. Once I had completed my rat studies, which demonstrated that sulphur-containing amino acids are essential for the nutritional benefits of the soybean, and had written my thesis, I had to defend my thesis in Muenster. After I had passed the last subject of the medical school examination, I officially became a physician. However, I could not practice in my own office until I had completed another fifteen months of internship.

My time in medical school was filled with interesting memories. Some were mundane and humorous—like the fact that we usually had running water, but no toilet paper. We used newspaper. And hot water was only rarely available, so we bathed with hot water only once weekly. We also wore our undergarments and shirts for several days in a row. I took my laundry to Aunt Kaetchen once every two to four weeks. But the American people provided clothing and food via many charitable organizations, CARE probably being the most known in Germany. The winter coat that I received in 1947 I used until leaving for America. But I also obtained ration coupons from German authorities to buy cheaply-made German clothing after the war.

There were no telephone connections between the Western Zone and the Russian Zone, despite the fact that Aunt Kaetchen in Willich, and my parents in Berlin, had telephones. I therefore could not talk to my parents. But I did write letters.

In a letter to Vati on August 3, 1946, I wrote that I was about to receive some of the things that the British soldiers had taken away from me in Muensterlager. This gave me more cigarettes and coffee to barter. Until 1948, prior to the currency reform, coffee, cigarettes, and chocolate were the most valuable bartering tools. One of the most basic items, however, was always in short supply. In my letters to relatives, I was always asking for writing paper. There was none in the West, but apparently there was some (poor quality) paper in the Russian Zone.

In the second semester, I had to be in Muenster the whole time. Classes were held every day except Friday. Sometime in the summer of 1946, I received, with the help of Uncle Max, a coupon to buy a bike. This bike was as important to me in Muenster as a car is today to most students. I always locked it up. At night I carried it into my living quarters several floors high. I remember I was once intoxicated on my way home from a party, and I fell off my bike in the center of town. A policeman came and helped me up, and I rode on.

At that time there were no private cars on the road, only British Army cars and trucks, and life on the street was safe. Another time I came home drunk from yet another party—remember, the alcohol consumed at that time was all homemade—I went to the room I had lived in previously, and carried my bike up two floors. I woke up my former landlord, and he must have sent me back to my current apartment, because when I woke up at noon the next day, I was in my new room, but without my bike. It took me a while to track my bike down to the place I lived before.

During the five years of study, I lived in at least four or five different places, renting rooms from different people. There were no apartments and no dormitories—just rooms for rent.

On August 1, 1946, we had a wonderful event in Buldern, about forty-five minutes by train from Muenster. It was held in a castle where many female students of the university lived. A female student whom I knew invited me as her guest. There were about forty couples in all at the grand party. The barracks where the students lived were on the grounds of a castle that belonged to the Baron von Blomberg. He contributed wine and strong beer; the British contributed several barrels of beer as well. We had all kinds of delicious food, including potato salad, bean salad, cheese, and so much more that one could not buy in Germany at that time. There was also a band and lots of dancing. The event lasted from eight o'clock in the evening until five-thirty the next morning (as determined by the availability of train transport home). The dean of the medical school and several professors were also there, as was the British university officer. The affair started with a polonaise, a stately formal dance for couples, through the whole castle.

Mr. Perraudin, the British university officer, came up to me during the festivities and asked me how my parents were doing. I told him that I was not allowed to travel to Berlin and had not seen them for more than three years. I then also told him that the food in the school cafeteria was very scarce, and that many students had difficulties with their studies because they were so hungry. Our German ration coupons assured us at the most 1,200 calories per day. It's true that there was not one really fat person at that time in all of Germany, and very few people experienced heart attacks. I learned early on that leanness and obesity are clearly influenced by calorie intake per day. While some people may metabolize their food faster than others, it still comes down to calories in, calories out. But too many of the students weren't getting enough calories. I hoped that the British could help by providing potatoes. He promised he would look into this matter. And he did.

Rebuilding Time

This was an interesting and often tense time in Germany's history. Despite my good experiences with Americans and the British, hatred against the Germans persisted in some circles, quite understandably, considering all that had gone on. US Secretary of the Treasury Morgenthau was among those who harbored a strong hatred of Germans. Long before the end of the war he proposed to tear down all the factories in Germany and make it an agrarian state. Yet Morgenthau's strongly-expressed opinion was not shared by President Roosevelt, or by much of mainstream America, and certainly not by President Truman, who took office when Roosevelt, already a sick man for several years, died. Winston Churchill, the British prime minister, believed Roosevelt had given up much too much to the Russian dictator, Stalin, at their meetings in Tehran and later in Yalta. And in fact, after the war ended, the Russians dismantled most of the unbombed factories in their zone, while the Western powers of America, England, and France did not do that in their zones.

What happened after the war was still amazing. Instead of hating the Germans, the Western allies, primarily America, helped Germany with its rebuilding. Even George Patton, the famous US general, turned friendly toward Germany after the end of the war. When he was killed in a car accident in Bavaria, rumor was that those allies who wanted to execute the Morgenthau plan had killed him. The American help to Germany, and later to all of Western Europe, is one of the greatest acts of modern charity, executed by the occupying forces of a victorious nation, who could just as easily have shown revenge. This assistance culminated in the Marshall Plan, announced by Secretary of State Marshall at Harvard in 1947.

General Marshall was head of the armed forces during the war and General Eisenhower's superior.

In late 1946 or early 1947, one simple word in the English language, used to convey something quite differently in Great Britain and America, caused Germans for months and months to eat cornbread instead of rye or wheat bread. When the Germans were asked what they needed most in food supplies, they responded with the German word *Korn,* referring to rye and wheat. However, the Americans interpreted this German word as corn, what the British call maize, and, in typical American efficiency, sent ships upon ships loaded with corn to Germany. This corn shipment kept thousands upon thousands of Germans alive after the war.

The Marshall Plan helped every country in Europe, including Germany. I later learned that in contrast to France and other countries, most Marshall Plan funds had to be returned to the German state within a certain period of time. In fact, some of the money was used many years later to integrate East Germany into West Germany after the wall came down in 1989.

Mr. Perraudin, the British university officer, extended some of that kindness toward Germany to me on a personal level. When I told him at the castle party that I hadn't yet visited my parents, he said, "We must do something about it. Please provide my office with your personal data and I will see what I can do." He then asked me to help him found an English Club at the university. I did, and the English Club remained active the whole time I was in Muenster. We held dinners and dances at the English Officers Club together with the military occupation forces and with students from other countries. The dinners always ended at midnight with everyone rising to their feet at the playing of the British national anthem.

I visited my grandmother (Oma), the mother of my father,

in Sande once per year, always at Pentecost. She was a warm and
wonderful person. She also was a supporter of my education and
regularly sent me a portion of her meager pension to help with my
school expenses. I took the daily express train from Muenster to
Wilhelmshaven, via Sande. Oma worked in her garden and did all
the cooking. Every time I visited, I always trimmed the big hedge
that separated her property from the neighbor's. It was a little too
much for her to cut. I also went with her to the Lutheran church
on Pfingsten.

In 1946, Oma's house was still partially occupied by the British. I lived with Aunt Gretel (Uncle Fritz's wife), but ate meals with
Oma. Uncle Fritz was a Nazi with the Golden party broche (only
the first 100,000 Nazis received this golden medal) and was still in
a Nazi internment camp. I felt that politically Aunt Gretel was also
still a Nazi.

I didn't speak about it, though, because I was worried about my
older cousin, Fritzi, who had been a soldier on the Russian front. I
wanted to help him study in Muenster, but he was listless and didn't
want to do anything. He just sat around for months at home, doing
nothing. Everyone was still waiting for Uncle Fritz to return.

Imme, his daughter, was quite different. She was in Moelle, Germany, married, and working in a British canteen. She later came to
Sande, and her first husband worked as a salesman for the homeo-
pathic pharmaceutical company, Madaus. One of their elixirs, Gold
Tropfen, contained ethyl alcohol and we made schnapps out of it.
In fact, until 1948, all liquor was made mostly from potatoes and in
secret alcohol mills, just as during the prohibition in America.

In late August 1946, Mr. Perraudin wrote to tell me I had to
go to my county seat, Kempen, and bring certification that I was
not a Nazi. After the war, all Germans had to go through a "de-

nazification" process. Since my father never belonged to the party, and neither did my relatives in Willich, who were all strict Roman Catholics, and because I never belonged to the Hitler Youth, and I completed the Fort Eustis Camp in the US, I had no problem with the "denazification" process.

After proving I wasn't a Nazi, I then completed a request form to travel to and from Berlin and brought it to the British Military Government in Muenster. He, Mr. Perraudin, promised to add his recommendation, and then forward the papers to the Control Commission in Berlin. He expected a response in two to three months.

Back to Berlin

Perhaps I should offer a brief explanation of how Germany was governed by the Allies after the war. Germany was divided into four territories, called zones. The Americans had most of southern Germany; the French had the southern area closest to France (it was the smallest zone); the British had northern and middle Germany; and the Russians governed the East. Berlin was an exception. It was governed by all four victorious countries. A commission consisting of the four allies ran Berlin, and the citizens of Berlin could travel freely within the whole city until the Russians finally built the Berlin Wall. They did this because many East Germans were fleeing the Russian Zone via Berlin.

As promised, I received my travel papers in November for travel to Berlin before Christmas with a return date of January 6 or 7, 1947. I took a train from Muenster to Hannover, and from there, a streetcar to the apartment of another British officer with whom I stayed overnight. In the morning his wife served me a typical British breakfast with fried eggs, fried tomatoes, bacon, and toast. The

British officer then drove me to the central train station and checked me into the British interzone train.

This train traveled once daily between the British zone and Berlin, and included a passenger car for German VIPs. All other cars were for British soldiers and officers. The train left Hannover late evening and arrived in Berlin the next morning. The Russians could only check our papers, nothing else, and that is why I had to have my papers; the Russians could not detain us.

When I arrived in Berlin for the first time in almost four years, I was shocked. Berlin was in ruins. My parents had been bombed out of their apartment, and luckily, after a few weeks, they were able to move into an apartment whose owner had left Berlin. Between apartments, my family lived for a few weeks in the candy factory where my father worked.

When I saw my parents and Gisela and Lothar for the first time in four years, I was so happy that they still were alive. My family had lost nearly everything when the apartment was bombed, other than a few things stored in the basement. But they were alive! After the Russian occupation of Berlin, my father was collected by the Russians and was supposed to be shipped to Siberia. Russian and Ukrainian civilians who had worked in his factory during the war went to the Russians and appealed to the authorities on my father's behalf.

"He treated us well," they said.

And because of their appeal, the Russians let my father go. Soon thereafter the factory was taken over by the Russians and converted from a war factory making lamps and war supplies, back again to a chocolate factory. This allowed my mother some bartering power in the black market, offering sweets for food and coal.

My parents invited Mr. Perraudin, my British friend, to join us for Christmas dinner on that first visit back to Berlin in 1946. He did, and we all had a great time. I also went with him to a couple of German theaters, one for Schiller's *Die Raeuber,* and I sat next to him and translated the dialogue during the show. Until Mr. Perraudin left Muenster in 1948 to return home, I kept up a close friendship with him. And he helped me whenever he could. But I made it a point not to appear as a beggar, but a friend, so I only reluctantly accepted gifts from him and always tried to do something for him in return.

On my return from this first Christmas trip I shared my train compartment with the future first German president, Dr. Theodor Heuss, and his staff. When under the Allies' oversight, (i.e. the Americans, British and French), a German government was elected. Dr. Adenauer, der Alte (the old one), the former mayor from Cologne, who was incarcerated by the Nazis, became chancellor of Germany as head of the Christian Democratic party, and Dr. Heuss was elected president. In the Russian Zone communists were placed into power and created a second, "independent," German state in the Russian Zone.

I visited my parents every Christmas from that first one on. From 1947 on, another daily train connected the British zone and Berlin, now only for Germans with special passes. The winters were usually very cold, particularly 1947 and 1948. When I woke up in the morning, the water in my washbasin was frozen. We had no coal to heat a room overnight. This was the same in Willich. On the floor where the bedrooms were, we had no heat and no bathroom. For emergencies we had a pot. Or, you could make the cold trek downstairs to the bathroom.

When Christmas 1948 came around, the interzone express was not running because of the Russian Berlin blockade. The Russians had blocked all traffic to Berlin, by train, by road, and by water (through canals and rivers). I took the train to Helmstedt, hoping to find transportation to Berlin. While I was looking around, a bus transporting children appeared from Bavaria. I went to the leader, a nurse, and told her that I was a young doctor and asked if she would allow me to take care of her sick children and accompany the transport. Everyone agreed, and I moved to the last row of the bus. None of us had to step out at the checkpoint, as the Russians did not want the children running around. Some Russians did enter the bus, but they didn't want to catch the illnesses and colds from the children, so they left the young doctor undisturbed.

To my parents' surprise, I arrived in Berlin. After the New Year, I went to the British authorities in Berlin and they gave me a pass to fly out to Hannover. I left Berlin in a three-engine, British coal-transport plane, sitting on the floor, covered by coal dust, but happy to get out of Berlin safely. We landed in Hannover, and I took a train home from there to Muenster. Meanwhile, President Truman stood up to the Russians, and after twelve months of blockades, the Russians caved in and again allowed traffic to Berlin. During the months of the complete blockade of Berlin from the free world, American and British supply planes landed every three minutes in their respective airports, Tempelhof and Gatow, providing Berlin with food and coal. This famous "Luft Bruecke" (airlift) kept Berlin alive.

The most exciting thing for me about this trip during the blockade was that my friend, Horst, a dental student whom I met in Muenster when I arrived in 1946, and who always believed he did everything better than anyone else, arrived one day later in Berlin. I had beaten him! We both left Muenster about the same time; he planned to sneak over the northern border close to Hamburg and Rostock.

My sister, Gisela, told me that the East German-communist government appeared several times a year at our apartment, picking up my father in a big Russian limousine to take him to their headquarters in Pankow, trying to persuade him to accept the post of minister of commerce for East Germany, as he was one of only a few non-Nazis in higher industry positions. But my father said, "I was able to avoid the Nazis, I will have to do the same now and avoid the Communists." And that's when my parents moved to West-Berlin.

Uncle Richard had returned from the war in 1947. He had an old motorbike that I borrowed after the currency reform, driving through the whole area of the state, selling Christmas and Easter candies for my father. By then, my father had left his factory, which the Russians had taken over, and moved to the American sector in Berlin. I think it was in about 1949 or 1950. He started to work for a former, much smaller, competitor, and when the wholesalers in West Germany heard that my father was running the show, they all ordered from me, and my sales profit supported part of my studies after 1948. In 1950 or 1951, before the Berlin Wall went up, my parents moved to Offenbach near Frankfurt to restart my father's old factory with the two sons of his former partner who didn't return from Russian captivity.

Shortly after I immigrated to the States, my poor father ran out of money and had to file for bankruptcy. He moved temporarily to Willich and lived with Aunt Kaetchen, working for an even smaller competitor in Krefeld. He later moved into the office building of this company and had a very nice apartment next to the factory. From there he was able, a few years later, to obtain an apartment on the Krefeld East Wall, a very nice living area in center city, and he worked in this position until he retired at age sixty-eight.

My mother, who in college earned a teaching degree, became

an elementary teacher, yet she had never taught until my parents moved to Krefeld. She worked from age fifty-five to sixty-eight. My mother primarily taught English, which she also spoke very well. She visited us many times in America, not only joining us for vacations, but also spending some time observing US teaching methods (and coming away impressed).

After the currency reform in West Germany in 1948, there was a brief window of time when I found a way to profit from the change. I bought German postal stamps in the Russian Zone with their useless money and then sold the same stamps in the West for the new good currency. This helped to carry me further in my studies, because after 1948 my parents' money was no help to me in the West.

I bought a few other things in the Russian sector with their useless money to re-sell in the West. Things like silk stockings, bras, and women's underwear that were being made in a former parachute factory. My friends always teased me that I offered the wares for less to pretty girls if they let me assist them in putting on the bras.

My parents really had a tough time financially, yet they were able to send their three children to medical school. Lothar, my younger brother, became a surgeon, eventually the chief surgeon in a large Catholic hospital in Witten, Ruhr Valley. Gisela, my sister, married Ahmad Agah, a Persian who studied medicine at the same university. Gisela and Ahmad were married in 1958 and started a large, general family practice in 1963 in Eschborn, a suburb of Frankfurt. After practicing for decades, their practice has since been taken over by two of their five daughters who also became doctors. But even now, Gisela, 78 years old, still practices a few half days per week.

Since it was difficult after the war for Germans to make contact with people from other countries, I took the opportunity that offered itself in the early summer of 1949 to work on a farm in Switzerland. Afterward, I hitchhiked all through Switzerland using the money earned on the farm, sleeping, if possible, in youth hostels. Hitchhiking was no problem at that time. A few female students in Muenster, who were war refugees from Estonia and Lithuania, kept records and collected attendance for practical studies and seminars at my university for me while I was away. It was a great experience. Switzerland was untouched by the war. American Cadillacs and other big US cars filled the streets. And while I lost something by skipping part of a semester in Muenster, I gained much from this enriching experience.

Crista

While in Muenster during the last two years of medical school I met Crista Loessin, whose father was of French Huguenot descent. One day, riding my bike through town, I saw Crista walking between lectures. I wanted to meet her, so I stopped my bike and talked to her. One thing led to another, and we started to date, and with time, fell in love.

Crista had also grown up in Berlin, in the suburb, Karlshorst. Crista was a rather shy, warm, and loving person. She was also very intelligent. At that time, she had just entered a PhD program in German and English literature.

In 1950, one did not even consider moving into a place together before being married. In addition, apartments for rent were not yet available in bombed out Germany; every student lived in furnished rooms. After a few years, Crista had to interrupt her studies for lack of funds, and started to work in another town as a secretary. Marriage was not yet possible, since I would have very little income

as an intern for the fifteen months after the completion of medical
school.

I took my final medical school examination during the tenth
semester between May and July 1951. One week later, and five
years after I entered medical school, I defended my MD dissertation. Then I spent my medical internship at three different places.
I worked as a volunteer at the X-ray Institute of Dr. Gerbaulet
in Duisburg. Dr. Gerbaulet was the brother-in-law of my friend,
Johann Kleist, whom I had met as a POW in the US and who had
arrived one year later than I, also in Muenster, to study law. I also
worked at the Institute of Hygiene in Dortmund, where my friend
Ulrich Loens' father was the director; and at the Medical Department of the city hospital of Dortmund. I still have contact with
Ulrich and his wife and visited him in 2009.

During the last year of my internship, I had a small apartment
in Dortmund. I was able to earn some income by doing blood
draws and syphilis tests at the institute of my friend's father. He was
famous as a paternity expert. I published my first scientific paper
on blood typing for paternity suits based on work I had done in
Dortmund.

After I had completed my internship, I got a job in Bamberg in
the city pathological institute run as a private enterprise by the chair
of microbiology at the University of Erlangen. Since Crista and I
wanted to get married, and we didn't want to live in Bamberg (the
laboratory was next to a slaughter house), I left Bamberg after a few
months. Life was still very tough in Germany. Medical internships
and most residencies paid nothing, or only very little. Crista's
mother and my parents were living under extremely difficult financial circumstances. So Crista and I had only a small family civil wedding in Dortmund before the city clerk in April 1953. A little later

we went by train to the Mosel River area for a short honeymoon and a religious wedding in a Catholic church.

Afterward, we moved in with my parents for three months while I, at the Institute of Pathology at Frankfurt University, learned to do autopsies. During these months I traveled to Frankfurt mostly by bike, but also by streetcar. I was able to obtain, partly through the help of my friend Ulrich's father, a paid assistantship in the large city hospital in Kassel, and I started to work in Kassel in July. Since I was influenced by my friend's father to join public health and pathology, this job, I hoped, would prepare me for a job in public health at Harvard, with which I corresponded at the time about a residency.

My main job was testing bacteria and their response to various antibiotics. But I also had the chance to participate in and do autopsies by myself. While in Kassel I was already into research and published three scientific papers. It is interesting that one of the papers dealt with the Agar Loch test, in which I could demonstrate that a given bacteria responded differently to antibiotics, depending on whether I first isolated the bacteria and tested the bacteria separately, or whether I tested them as a mixed culture as they grew in the human body. At that time, psychiatry was the farthest thing from my mind, yet I was interested in the interaction of bacteria with antibiotics. There was only one small step to become interested in studying the interaction between various treatments in psychiatry and what I later described as nonspecific factors in a treatment situation.

Finally earning a halfway decent salary, we were able to move into a small apartment in Kassel in the private house of a woman whose brother was a Jesuit priest and active in helping Germans emigrate to America. (This, however, we learned only later.) Crista took the job of secretary to a CEO of a big company, the name of which I have forgotten. Kassel was a nice town, severely damaged during the war, but already being rebuilt. It had a big park on a hill, with waterfalls running down, and a castle on the top. On Sundays there were big water fountain displays.

After being at Kassel for fewer than six months, I saw an ad in a German medical journal offering sponsorship to emigrate to the United States if I would commit myself to spend at least one year at the Mental Health Institute of Cherokee, Iowa. Apparently, at that time, psychiatrists were in short supply in America, at least in state hospitals. The proposed sponsor was a Swedish farmer couple by the name of Gustafson. I started my application process at once, and since our institute did all the bacteriological examinations of blood specimens for the US Army hospital, I always had a place on a US Army truck going to Frankfurt when I needed to go to the US Consulate to promote our visa applications.

In the meantime, Crista had become pregnant with our son, Larry. We were worried that the mental hospital in America would not take us because of her pregnancy, so we didn't tell them. We were also worried that the visa application might draw out so long that Crista could not travel, and we would have to stay in Germany. After a few more trips to the US Consulate in Frankfurt, I was finally able to obtain visas for Crista and me. Emigration to America was not an easy step for either of us emotionally, but Crista supported me wholeheartedly.

We were terribly excited to be able to emigrate to America. Times were still very difficult in Germany, and particularly for someone who wanted to go into academia and research. We saw this as an opportunity for our family and my future career. But most importantly, ever since my time as a POW in America, I knew that I wanted to return to this wonderful country permanently.

Thanks to our landlord's brother, a Jesuit priest who provided transportation for emigrants through the Catholic charity, we were able to get inexpensive tickets on a turbo prop charter plane (jets did not yet fly commercially). The flight took us from Frankfurt to Prestwick, Scotland; Reykjavik, Iceland; Gander, Newfoundland; and finally, New York. It was a long trip, about twenty- five hours of travel time, but we made it. It was thrilling to finally arrive in America, but we were also tired and worried about the stress of travel on Crista and the baby. It was the first of September 1954, when, for the second time, I landed on American soil. My dream of a new home was fulfilled.

The German Jesuit priest also provided us a hotel room in New York for a few days, a plane ticket from New York to Chicago, and the night train ticket to Cherokee, Iowa. The morning of September 10, 1954, we arrived in Cherokee and were welcomed by several physicians from the hospital. The next day, I began my life as a psychiatrist. I was 30 years old at the time. Ever since the Jesuit priest helped me and Crista to emigrate to the United States, I have been supporting the Catholic charity, irrespective of whether we attended the Catholic or Episcopal church.

4

America Becomes Home

Everyone was surprised when they met Crista, very much pregnant, but they didn't turn us away. In fact, the hospital gave us a nice apartment on the grounds. Larry was born on December 2, 1954, in the small local hospital, delivered by the only general practitioner in town. Soon after we arrived in Cherokee I bought a four-year-old Buick Roadmaster for $900. That car was one of only two things I ever bought with borrowed money. The other was a sewing machine from Sears for Crista.

Everyone in Cherokee was very nice to us. There were several immigrants at the hospital, Germans primarily. Our sponsor family, the Gustafsons, was awfully nice. Like the rest of the people we met, they were hard-working, Lutheran, and God-fearing people. Most families in Cherokee were of Scandinavian and northern German descent. The experience we had in Iowa showed us that Middle America was quite different than the East Coast.

When I arrived at Cherokee State Hospital in September 1954, I was impressed by its cleanliness and the surrounding acreage where patients worked on a farm and in a tree nursery. But when visiting the closed wards of the hospital, I became keenly aware of the ineffectiveness of psychiatric treatment at the time. Here, violent schizophrenic patients sat in restraints consisting of large leather contraptions.

Before Psychopharmacology

It was still a time in psychiatry when barbiturates and bromides, the only sedatives available, did not work, and straightjackets, cold water baths, electroshock therapy, insulin shock, and transorbital lobotomy were the treatments used to control violent, aggressive, but also just very unruly, patients. But the hospital was definitely not a "snake pit," as so many mental facilities were described at that time.

The diagnoses of the patients were primarily schizophrenia, manic-depressive illness, and severe forms of epilepsy, plus an assortment of rare mental disorders such as "Huntington's chorea." Occupational and social therapies were the main treatment methods of mental patients at that time. Most patients worked on the hospital farm and got frequent passes to visit their relatives.

There was ample support staff, primarily nurses and big, strong orderlies. The hospital also had a well-run medical ward and an outpatient infirmary. The only general practitioner in town made medical rounds occasionally, while the psychiatric staff, mostly immigrants, not yet board-eligible, took care of both the psychiatric and medical needs of our patients. The superintendent, who was probably the only non-immigrant, ran the hospital, assisted by two medical directors, both refugees from Nazi occupation who had trained in Germany. Each physician was responsible for several patient wards. Patients were housed in open wards that held thirty to forty beds each. The medical staff, nurses, and orderlies all had good relationships with each other.

Electroshock therapy, also called electroconvulsive therapy, or ECT, was used to temporarily lower the aggressive, destructive behavior of chronically psychotic patients. At that time electroshock was given with Anectin, a muscle relaxant, to prevent the frequent lumbar and thoracic compression fractures that occurred with the ECT-induced grand mal convulsions. Since the muscle relaxant also affected the chest muscles, patients had difficulty breathing, and were given oxygen during and after the treatment. Until patients lost consciousness during electroshock, they sometimes felt like they were suffocating. There was no anesthetist, and therefore no sedation. Usually, ten or more patients received treatment, one after the other, in the same room. Today ECT is given under anesthesia and sedation. Insulin shock treatment was given much less frequently; it was much more involved and needed a large amount of staff supervision.

Another approach to helping violent patients was transorbital lobotomy, developed by the neurologist, Dr. Freeman, who was the uncle of a friend of mine. Twice monthly, a neurologist (it could have been Dr. Freeman himself) came to the hospital and performed these lobotomies, and taught one of our medical directors how to perform the procedure. Patients were anesthetized via ECT, and then an ice pick was pushed into the frontal lobe with entry above the eyeballs. Once the ice pick was in the frontal cortex, several medial and lateral movements were made with the purpose of cutting connections from the frontal lobe to other parts of the brain.

The result was, indeed, a rather placid, much more manageable patient. Several lobotomies were done at the same time. I believe consent was usually obtained from the family beforehand. But keep in mind, institutional review boards and informed consent procedures did not yet exist. Critics argued that the transorbital lobotomy only created vegetables. This wasn't true. One has to remember that without the benefits of transorbital lobotomies, such patients would have to be kept constantly in restraint. I believe it was a helpful option at that time.

While in Cherokee, I was introduced to the American sport and entertainment of wrestling. I visited Sioux City, about an hour away from Cherokee, to see my first wrestling matches. Once in Philadelphia, I visited a few more matches in the Arena on Market Street, a sports hall which was torn down about ten years later.

The Beginnings of Psychopharmacology

I had been in Cherokee a few months when we were able to obtain large amounts of samples of the first two antipsychotic drugs ever developed, chlorpromazine (Thorazine) and reserpine (Serpasil), from Smith Kline & French Laboratories in Philadelphia, and from Ciba, Switzerland, respectively. Suddenly, patients who had been violent and aggressive for many years were quiet and controllable. They could dress themselves, eat on their own, and no longer soiled themselves. The stench that had been pervasive on the wards where these violent patients lived disappeared. It was truly a wonder.

Clearly, in the next few years, these and other drugs of the same class would revolutionize the treatment of psychotic patients all over the world, replacing transorbital lobotomy, insulin shock, and, to a large extent, electroshock therapy. However, even today, ECT is still often the treatment of last resort in severely depressed patients. In fact, when I came to the Hospital of the University of Pennsylvania (HUP) in September 1955, we still had a number of depressed patients who were well-maintained receiving outpatient ECT once monthly.

Once I had been in Cherokee for about six months, I decided that psychiatry, not public health and pathology, was my calling. Psychiatry stood at a crossroads. A new type of treatment, namely the potential use of clinically effective medications to treat psychiatric illnesses, had appeared from nowhere. I wanted to be involved in this revolutionary development from its beginning, and hoped to become an important player in this new field.

Because of this, I wanted to obtain further training. I applied to Harvard, the University of Pennsylvania (Penn), and Johns Hopkins, the only three places I knew on the East Coast where I would consider learning. (I didn't want to live and work in New York.) Penn called me and said they just might have an opening, and asked if I could come for an interview. I said that I would love to enter their residency, but if I would visit them now, I would have no money to start my residency. They gave me an interview over the telephone.

Dr. Emily Mudd conducted most of the interview. Dr. Mudd was a protégé of Dr. Kenneth Appel, chair of Penn's department of psychiatry, and head of the Philadelphia Marriage Council, with whom I later collaborated in women's health. I believe Penn wanted me in their residency because of my three German scientific publications. They wanted someone with an interest in research.

When I'd been at Penn for a few years, Dr. Mudd told me that they did contact my superintendent at Cherokee for a reference. His response was, "As an immigrant, he is okay, but not the quality of an American medical school graduate." So they asked him, "We can assume, then, that you are going to let him go soon?" to which he replied, "Oh, no, we definitely want to keep him here." Penn then realized that he was giving me a bad recommendation to keep me. And so they hired me.

We liked it in Cherokee, but I was getting restless and wanted to move on. I had learned all that Cherokee had to offer me. I was very much looking forward to receiving the best training America had to offer, and was looking for a good place to further my training and career. Training in psychotherapy of psychiatric patients was my goal, and so we soon began making preparations for a move to Philadelphia.

Penn Beckons

After my year in Cherokee ended on September 12, 1955, I packed the Buick with Crista, Larry, and our few belongings, and we headed to Philadelphia. The day we arrived I found, through the hospital, a furnished apartment in West Philadelphia on 44th and Baltimore. We stayed there for about one year, cooled not by a fan, but a window air conditioner purchased from one of the discount stores on Frankfurt Avenue in Northeast Philadelphia.

We exchanged the Buick for an inexpensive black Studebaker with red, fake-leather upholstery. It was a make that soon thereafter went bankrupt. The summer of 1956, one year after we had arrived at Penn, Dr. Appel let us use his farmhouse in New Hampshire for a week-long vacation. It had no heat, but many fireplaces and lots of firewood to warm the cool nights. We had a great time, and also visited Concord and the White Mountains. Another summer we spent a September week at the New Jersey shore. It reminded me of the Baltic, where I spent many summers with my parents. We had a great time.

It didn't take too long for Crista to tire of the furnished apartment. She found us a garden apartment in Drexel Brook, where we lived for the next several years. It had two bedrooms, one bath, a living/dining room, and one window air conditioner. My yearly income as a fellow was $2,800, but Dr. Appel gave me additional funds for attending several biological psychiatry meetings, keeping notes for him, and updating him on my return. I was thankful for the additional opportunity, but I'm convinced that Dr. Appel just wanted to help Crista and me.

Our residency program was small and elite. We were six second-year fellows in the program, two each from Texas and Pennsylvania, and one each from California and Germany. Our training basically focused on psychoanalysis and psychoanalytic psychotherapy. Dr. Appel spent each day until noon teaching and running the department from the Functional Clinic at the Hospital of the University of Pennsylvania (HUP). In the afternoon he ran a large private practice at Forty-Ninth Street, or the "Institute," as it was called. It was one of the most famous psychiatric institutions in America. All the leading psychiatrists and analysts in the city practiced there, and Dr. Appel always had a group of psychiatric associates working for him. It was no wonder that my meetings with Dr. Appel usually took place, not at HUP, but at the Institute, after he had seen his last private patient, which was often around midnight.

The Institute had both inpatients and outpatients. It was located in West Philadelphia on large grounds in a palatial setting. Psychotic members of the most famous and rich families of Philadelphia, the Main Line, and Wilmington, Delaware—but also from all over the United States—lived there for many years, some even for their whole lives. The Institute does not exist anymore, as it had outlived its usefulness. Medication treatment, as well as subtypes of psychotherapy, such as cognitive and interpersonal psychotherapy and behavior therapy, largely replaced psychoanalysis and psycho-analytic therapy. Hospitalization today is usually for much shorter periods of time than in the 1950s and 1960s. Psychoanalysis primarily exists merely as a theory of personality. It still serves in the teaching of our residents of how best to understand the emotional make-up of their patients, and of human behavior in general.

During my residency I was given some time for more basic research, and Christian Lambertsen, MD, professor of pharmacology, became my first research mentor, and later my personal friend. I still remember his advice: "When you present a paper, try to get only one, or in rare cases, two messages across. If you do more, your listeners will lose you." I tried to follow his advice, but sometimes I failed, compelled as I was by the strong desire to communicate all of my findings. I must admit that I have this tendency even today.

Under Dr. Lambertsen's guidance I conducted a study testing the differential effects of various anticonvulsant drugs in monkeys in whom convulsion was introduced by the administration of carbon dioxide. I presented the results of this study, my first study conducted as a resident, at the Federation Proceedings of 1958, and an abstract was published. In the next year, again at the Federation Proceedings, I presented data on the cold pressure test, which measured blood pressure and heart rate in response to placing one hand into a bucket of ice water, and the results from which differentiated between anxious and non-anxious patients. It was later published in a psychiatric journal. One of the meetings was in Atlantic City and one in Chicago, to which I traveled by sleeper train. The Federation Proceedings was the largest annual scientific meeting at that time.

Another project I worked on as a resident involved giving anxious patients, on alternate weeks, inhalations of either carbon dioxide or nitrous oxide. We studied the patients' response under each gas, the sensory constants occurring during gas inhalation, dreams under inhalation and at home, and the free associations to both types of dreams. The use of these drug inhalations was hoped to facilitate psychotherapy. Regretfully, the data was never published. The final project I was involved in with Dr. Lambertsen was the study of cerebral blood flow in schizophrenic patients at the Delaware State Hospital. Most important for me at that time was that I received fifty dollars for the morning we spent in Delaware. This supported my meager university salary.

Lessons from a Mentor

Dr. Appel was a great man who was adored by his patients and co-workers. I learned a lot from him. In one of my earliest supervisory sessions with Dr. Appel, I remarked that a psychotherapy patient for whom I had prescribed the barbiturate, Alurate, to help him with his anxiety, complained to me that its efficacy was decreasing. Dr. Appel reminded me that Alurate was available in two colors, pink and green, and told me to prescribe the other color for the patient. And, indeed, the patient responded to the same medication in a different color. This demonstrated to me how the power of persuasion and expectation could influence the patient's response to medication.

There is another supervisory session I had with Dr. Appel I will never forget. I had examined a female patient in her forties for fifty minutes and had gotten nowhere. Dr. Appel came in and joined us and asked the patient not about possible symptoms or why she came to the clinic, but simply about her life. Her face lit up and she told him that she was a part-time Avon sales lady. Dr. Appel asked her what products she had with her, and on the spot he bought something for Mrs. Appel. Within ten minutes he found out what events led to her being sent to the clinic. He had established a patient-psychiatrist relationship with her. During the whole interview, which probably did not last for more than fifteen minutes, total, Dr. Appel held constant eye contact with the patient, expressing caring and warmth, even holding her hand a few times. That amazed me and served as one of the most important examples of how I wanted to act and treat my patients.

Let me talk for a minute about our hospital consultation service. Residents usually did consultation at the hospital in the morning, and saw psychotherapy patients in the afternoon, as well as on Thursday evenings and on Saturday mornings. Since my co-residents were all psychoanalytically oriented, their consultation notes dealt with psychoanalytic interpretation of the patient's problem, but very little with practical recommendation of what to do with the patient for the few days that he was in the hospital. In contrast, I was pragmatic in my approach, and, therefore, my recommendations were liked by internists, general surgeons, and orthopedic surgeons alike.

For example, one patient I saw was an elderly orthopedic patient who appeared confused and had to be restrained to his bed. I recommended a night-light and a few pictures of children and grandchildren be placed on the nightstand. His confusion cleared up at once. Another time I was called to a non-English-speaking, supposedly psychotic, patient. When I visited him at his bed, he seemed to focus on his lower abdomen. When I examined him, he had a tremendously distended bladder. My treatment recommendation was to catheterize the patient's bladder.

The Birth of Psychopharmacology

From the early fifties to the middle sixties psychiatric drugs entered the market in rapid succession, some to compete with meprobamate (Miltown) for the treatment of anxiety, and others, particularly

the anti-psychotics, to take market share away from chlorpromazine (Thorazine) in the treatment of psychotic illness. Thus, the
newly established Psychopharmacology Service Center of the National Institute of Mental Health (NIMH), under the leadership of
a young psychiatrist, Jonathan Cole, organized a three-day meeting at NIMH in September 1956. Cole was spending two years at
the Public Health Service as part of his draft requirement. In this
meeting, for the very first time, NIMH brought together scientists,
psychiatrists, pharmacologists, physiologists, sociologists, and psychologists, who were interested in this new field.

Since I was still a resident, I didn't participate. At that time
great interest existed in hallucinogenic drugs (such as LSD and
mescaline) to induce psychotic symptoms. Researchers hoped to
use these drugs to facilitate psychotherapy, but also to test antipsychotic drugs in such subjects. Even the army was greatly interested
in this work. The meeting attendants included researchers involved
in pain, sleep, stress, laboratory, and psychiatric research, the latter
primarily with inpatients.

The new NIMH Psychopharmacology Service Center received
several million dollars from the US Congress, a great sum of money
at that time, to stimulate research in Psychopharmacology. Thus,
right after my residency in late 1957, I prepared my first grant application to NIMH to study drug treatment in neurotic outpatients.

At that time, and until at least the mid-1980s when I was a
member of one of the NIMH peer review groups from 1977 to
1981, the NIMH research grants were reviewed according to the
following process: a grant application was submitted, and if it seemed
worthy to the program staff and principal reviewer, a site visit was
arranged, which usually included one NIMH staff person and at
least two members of the review panel.

That's exactly what happened with my first grant proposal. I remember only one of the three persons who visited me, Dr. Heinz Lehmann from Montreal, at that time one of the leading clinical psychiatrists and psychopharmacologists in North America. He had introduced chlorpromazine (Thorazine) for the treatment of schizophrenia and later imipramine (Tofranil) for the treatment of depression into the American continent, as he was one of only a few Canadian psychiatrists who spoke both French and English fluently. Dr. Lehmann was psychiatrist-in-chief at Verdun State Hospital in Montreal, where he lived all his life in a private home on the grounds of the hospital. During the visit, Dr. Lehmann and I were surprised to find out that his father, an eye, ear, nose, and throat (EENT) specialist in Berlin, had taken my adenoids out in the early 1930s. It is indeed a small world.

I got my first grant with my first submission. I feel fortunate that nearly all of my grant applications to NIMH, made over the past 50 years, were funded the first time around. The only exception was my last one, a six-year grant studying the role of long-term treatment of anxiety with medication, which took me three submissions to NIMH before receiving funding. The study started in January 2004 and ended December 31, 2009.

But before this, starting at the end of my last year of residency, I planned and conducted the first, or at least one of the earliest, placebo-controlled, double-blind, outpatient studies with anxious medical clinic outpatients. My collaborators were internists, not psychiatrists. I had to go to the HUP medical outpatient clinic because psychiatrists in the psychiatric clinic refused me access to their patients. Drugs simply were not used in a psychoanalytic clinic. But Dr. Appel, my mentor, encouraged me to go ahead.

This taught me another valuable lesson. *If you believe in what you want to do, do not give up.* Go to the person in charge. Such a person usually is in charge because he or she has more wisdom than the people reporting to them. They also are more open-minded. In later years, when I was a consultant to pharmaceutical firms, I only accepted such a relationship when I had an open door to the CEO and the vice president of research.

The medical clinic had many patients who were neurotic, in other words, anxious, and were receiving no treatment or, at the most, barbiturates. The study was done without any support other than my meager resident salary. The medication, however, was provided to us by Smith Kline & French Laboratories and Wallace Laboratories, and was double-blinded by the HUP pharmacy. Using a crossover design, the study compared the anti-anxiety drug meprobamate (Miltown), the antipsychotic drug prochlorperazine (Compazine), used in a low dosage also for anxiety, and amobarbital (Amytal), a barbiturate frequently used in anxious outpatients, with placebo in the same patient.

Up to this time, none of these three medications had ever been tested against a placebo. The medications were given in random order to fifty-one patients, and the results demonstrated efficacy of meprobamate over placebo, with amobarbital and prochlorperazine assuming an intermediary position in terms of efficacy. Only meprobamate (Miltown) produced significantly more clinical improvement than placebo. The results of this controlled trial were published in one of the leading medical journals, the *Journal of the American Medical Association* (*JAMA*), in 1959. Research methodology was still in its infancy. Clinical research methodology and placebo controls were first employed in pain research after the war. The Cornell Conference in 1947 was, I believe, the first conference held with the main focus on the placebo response.

One of my mentors at that time was Jim Ewing, a psychoanalyst with interest in psychopharmacology. From 1958 to 1961, we co-authored a yearly review chapter entitled "Drugs in Psychiatry" for the Davis Cyclopedia of Medicine, one of the premier treatment updates for the whole of medicine at that time. These chapters reflect the tremendously swift introduction of new psychiatric medications in the early period of psychopharmacology.

In our 1958 chapter, we had only a few drugs to discuss, mainly several antipsychotics, the anxiolytic Miltown, and one antidepressant (Marsalid). In 1959 we first mentioned imipramine (Tofranil), the first tricyclic antidepressant which was still in the drug-testing phase. In 1960 we mentioned the experimental drug RO5-0690 (Librium) as a most promising new minor tranquilizer. We only talked about efficacy and safety, as the mechanism of action of Librium was not yet known. In fact, its mechanism was discovered only in the late 1970s. Iproniazid (Marsilid) had by then been largely replaced by three less toxic monamine oxidase inhibitors (MAOI), and the anti-depressant imipramine got high praises from many authors.

Our last chapter in this series, which now covered far more than fifty medications, pointed out that the rauwolfia derivatives (Serpasil) were losing clinical favor as antipsychotics and were largely replaced by the phenothiazines, such as Thorazine, Compazine and Stellazine, that Librium had officially entered the market as an anti-anxiety drug, and that Valium was not far behind, both belonging to the class of benzodiazepines.

At the end of my residency in September 1957, Dr. Appel, a man I respected so much I was never able to address him by his first name, offered me a staff position in research for two years with the expectation that by that time I would bring in my own research funds. He advised me not to waste my time getting psychoanalytic training, which all my co-residents did. Dr. Appel said, "Karl, you will be an expert in this new field of biological psychiatry in no time, and the whole world will recognize you as an expert! You will become famous and rich."

As I considered Dr. Appel not only my mentor, but also a father figure, I followed his advice and did as he had recommended. I never regretted it. I continued to receive uninterrupted peer-reviewed NIMH research funding from 1959 to 2009.

However, influenced by my academic psychoanalytic elders, who advised me not to go into clinical psychopharmacology, but to study the physiological indicators of anxiety, a more academic and scientific area of research according to them, I also spent some time testing patients with a polygraph, assessed the Hypuric Acid Index as a measure of anxiety, and studied the cold pressure and methacholine tests as indicators of autonomic reactivity.

While academically interesting, I realized that physiology research did not promise me an exciting future, and it certainly would not lead me to help my patients with newly discovered treatments. Thus once I had my first ever outpatient study published in *JAMA*, and had obtained my first NIMH grant in 1959, I left the physiology of anxiety and stress and decided to become an expert in the pharmacological treatment of anxious and depressed neurotic outpatients.

Settling Into Life and Work

In the midst of all this work, Crista and I were traveling a lot and were also looking for a place to settle. We visited Eagles Mere in 1959 or 1960, which is located in the Endless Mountains of Pennsylvania, about three hours from our house. We stayed at the Forrest Inn, a property surrounded by sixty cottages, one of which was owned by a neighbor who recommended the town as a vacation spot. As was usual at that time, dinner for men was in jacket and tie, and naturally, there was no air conditioning.

At night we visited the town dump to watch the black bears search for food. It was a surreal scene, lit only by the headlights of parked cars. The Eagles Mere spring-fed lake is at an elevation of 2,000 feet and is surrounded by a trail through laurel, rhododendron, and pine trees. It reminded us at that time of an Indian path. Right in front of the hotel was a sandy beach area, just like at the New Jersey shore, only much, much smaller. The hotel was closed in the 1970s and torn down in the 1990s, but the cottages are still there. What a surprise when my son, Mike, and his wife, Alyssa, decided to buy a cottage in Eagles Mere seven years ago.

In 1960, Crista found us a home in Gladwyne. We were somewhat surprised when they asked us if we were Jewish. Apparently, the real estate sales people in Gladwyne did not yet show houses to Jewish people. Once again, we'd encountered evidence of prejudice. It was a curious time in America, to be sure.

Later in 1960, Crista, Larry, and I visited Mexico City so I could present one of the first papers on the new tranquilizer, Librium. On the way we stopped in Dallas to visit one of my fellow psychiatrists who had spent two years of residency with me. We also spent a few days in Acapulco.

For me, psychiatry was becoming more and more exciting. I entered psychiatry at the end of an era when occupational therapy and social management were the main treatments for psychotic patients in state mental institutions, while in private mental hospitals psychoanalysis was the treatment of choice. Psychoanalysis was the holy grail of psychiatric treatment. But none of these treatment options seemed to be truly effective.

The psychiatric scene was not much better for neurotic outpatients. Psychoanalysis, or psychoanalytic psychotherapy, was the only acceptable treatment in America and was rather ineffective. Most chairs of psychiatric departments were psychoanalysts, which was quite in contrast to Europe, where psychoanalysis originated. American psychiatry was resistant to the introduction of drugs for the treatment of mental illness. For anxiety, the new wonder drug, Miltown, had proven successful in many patients, but was mostly prescribed by non-psychiatrists, mainly family practice physicians or internists. Academia had very little use for Miltown, or, later, for Librium and Valium, in the treatment of neurotic disorders other than, at times, facilitating psychotherapy. And even so, many analysts maintained their belief that drug use, when combined with psychotherapy, was detrimental to the psychotherapeutic process. Miltown was introduced in 1955 at a New York meeting by Aldous Huxley. It became famous after the TV comedian, Milton Berle, said on his TV show that he would change his name from "Milton to Miltown" because the medication helped him so much.

So, it is no wonder that psychopharmacology, the treatment of the psyche with pharmacological agents, started out and grew in the large state mental hospitals and not at academic centers. Some state mental institutions also had small research centers, while others did not. Rockland State Hospital is a good example of those state institutions that had such a research center. The center was directed by the psychiatrist, Nathan Kline, who also had a large Manhattan private practice. Thus, US leaders in the field came from the state hospital system or from pharmacology.

I am not convinced that it was a good idea to close so many of the state hospitals with the goal to treat mental patients as outpatients. This is particularly true because the cities and states did not provide enough financial funds to support mental health treatment. For example, I believe that many patients at Cherokee were better off than patients treated today in community mental health centers. The fact is that even with all the new drugs we have available today, cure rates are still rather low. Some schizophrenic patients today end up in prisons or homeless on the street.

After my residency was over, in September 1957, I started to see private patients. By 1958, we had saved enough money to return to Germany for the first time. Crista, Larry, and I flew to Brussels, Belgium, where the World's Fair of 1958 was held, and where we slept in barracks set up for fair visitors. Then we spent a few days in Paris, where we stayed in a lovely old hotel. From Paris we flew to Switzerland, where we rented a car and drove for ten days all over Switzerland; Larry was just four at that time.

From Zurich I flew to Rome and attended the Collegium Internationale Neuro-Psychopharmacologicum (CINP) congress, while Crista and Larry flew to be with her mother and sister in Gelsenkirchen-Buer, Germany. At that time I always wore washable suits. And when I was in Rome, the congress arranged for an excursion to Tivoli Gardens, where a little Italian boy jumped into a pool of dirty water, spraying me all over. This was my only suit, and I had to give my paper the next morning. I washed my suit that evening and hung it up over the bathtub to dry. When I wore it the next morning for my presentation, it was still not only damp, but wet.

In 1960 I flew to Basel, Switzerland for the CINP congress, stopped to see my parents in Krefeld, and also visited Willich. I picked up a VW Beetle in Dusseldorf and shipped it home after my visit. Back then, it was cheaper to buy German cars in Germany and ship them to America. I went to Basel from Krefeld by train along the Rhine.

The next year, Crista, Larry, and I visited Copenhagen and Stockholm, where I participated in a symposium on benzodiazepines at a World Congress of Pharmacology. We stayed at the new Sheraton in Stockholm, had the official congress dinner at the city hall, and later visited Tivoli, an entertainment and amusement park in the center of Copenhagen, but also visited a nightclub with a very risqué show.

We did some traveling within the United States around Easter of 1961, driving by car to Florida. On the way, we stopped for a few days at the Williamsburg Inn, visiting Williamsburg and Jamestown, and then drove to North Carolina. When we finally got to Florida, we visited Cypress Gardens (a destination resort in the middle of Florida—Disney World did not yet exist), then continued on to Miami, where we stayed for a few days on the beach. We then returned to Philadelphia via St. Augustine, Charleston, and Virginia Beach. We enjoyed these trips, but it always felt good when we finally arrived home.

During these early years in Philadelphia, we started to adjust to our new country. We made many new friends at work and through Larry's Gladwyne Elementary School, and also got to know our neighbors. Crista resumed her PhD studies in English literature at Villanova University.

When Larry was born, we had him baptized Catholic. But later, since Crista was Lutheran and I was Catholic, we came to a compromise and joined the Episcopalian church in Gladwyne.

Penn's department of psychiatry was rather small at that time and many of its leading members were nationally recognized clinicians. Dr. Appel gave a yearly cocktail party for the whole department, which truly impressed Crista and me. Dr. Appel had severe arthritis in his hips and must have lived with constant pain. He was constantly walking with crutches (this was before replacement surgery had become common). Yet he always had a smile, a positive and warm disposition. He was the leader everyone wanted to emulate.

Crista's Cancer

In early summer 1962, while swimming at a small pool in Gladwyne, Crista noticed abdominal pain. She was operated on shortly thereafter in June 1962. An ovarian cyst was suspected, but the doctors instead discovered ovarian cancer. It had already spread. Though Crista's prognosis was considered very poor, we were advised not to cancel our planned European trip. Her doctors hoped that Crista might enjoy what could possibly be the last trip in her life.

Crista, Larry, and I traveled to Europe on the RMS Queen Mary to Le Havre, then visited Mont St. Michelle at the French Channel coast and other places in southern France, northern Italy, Switzerland, and several places in Germany, including Berlin. I don't remember much about our trip, as I was deeply upset and worried about Crista. I do recall we had our American car with us, and that we visited Amsterdam for a few days. Larry spent part of the summer with Crista's sister, Ursula, and her family, camping. We tried our best to enjoy the trip, but it was tough for both of us. The doctors' words proved prophetic: it would be our last vacation together. I tried to make the trip as wonderful an experience for Crista as possible, and we tried to enjoy every moment.

Through a friend, we consulted with the chair of OB-GYN in Cologne, and he confirmed that the tumor had already spread. We returned to the US from Paris on Pan Am, while our car was shipped home. Crista's mother came with us to America to help her daughter and our family. She was a wonderful support, but it must have been very tough for her to see her youngest daughter get sicker and sicker. I have repressed a lot about that period of my life because it was so painful.

Crista went through several operations, chemotherapy, and radiation therapy, but died about nine months after the cancer had been detected; Crista was only 37 years old. Six weeks prior to her death, in February 1963, Crista and I gave a small cocktail party in honor of her sister Ursula, who was visiting. A close friend took Ursula for a day trip to New York. All our friends were great and supportive of Crista and me. They also accompanied Crista to her radiation treatments.

Here was Crista, a young and beautiful woman and mother, who was willing to live with me through thick and thin until we reached our goal and had established ourselves in America. I was a workaholic then (and since), working late hours and even in the evening after I got home. When we were finally settled, and Crista could enjoy a good life, suddenly it was over. I was devastated.

After Crista had passed away, one of our friends, the wife of one of my fellow residents, was most helpful and took over all arrangements for the funeral. I was in a complete fog. I will never forget seeing Crista at the funeral home during the open casket viewing. She was all made up with powder and lipstick—I was shocked! This was not the memory that Larry or I wanted. I never dared to ask Larry about his reaction. The funeral was held at St. Christopher Church in Gladwyne, and many friends, colleagues, and acquaintances, even my collaborators from Hopkins and Washington, came. This was the only open casket viewing I ever attended in my life.

102 A Serendipitous Life

One of Crista's greatest desires was that Larry would be brought up in America and in a caring home. He was a sensitive young boy. I promised Crista that I would not let her sister raise Larry in Germany, that I would raise him. But I also promised Crista that I would encourage Larry to spend every summer with her sister and her family in Germany. Crista died much too young in April 1963. Her mother, Ellie, was with us to take care of Larry and me. Larry was barely eight years old.

A Fateful Trip

Soon after Crista's death, I went to Europe for eight weeks to try to come to grips with my loss. Oma Ellie and Larry had traveled earlier, as soon as school was over. During the summer Larry and I spent some time together and went to a meeting in Prague. It was at the height of the Cold War. When I was finally able to rent a car for two days to visit Karlsberg Castle with Larry, we were astounded that every person we encountered tried to stay away from us. We finally found out that the license plate on our rental car was recognized as a secret police license plate. Another interesting observation we made was that older people spoke a little German as their second language and the younger people, English.

Later we also visited England and its environment; I had rented a car, which I slightly smashed up. Then we drove to the south of England after visiting London. There we met up with a friend to sail in the Channel at South Devon. Larry spent the rest of the summer with the family of Crista's sister, and I with my family. On the plane on our way home from Paris, Crista's mother, Ellie, and Larry and I met a young woman named Linda and her three brothers and their parents.

We were sitting just one row apart.

Crista's mother, Ellie, Larry, and I sat in one row together in economy class. The planes in those days were rarely full and there were a number of rows completely free. The same summer Linda and her family had been on a European trip together and were on their way home to Pitman, New Jersey. They began the flight a couple of rows back. But once the plane was in the air, Linda and one of her brothers moved two rows forward into the empty row next to ours. It was then that Linda and I noticed each other.

Linda was going back to Salem College in Winston-Salem, North Carolina, where she was a senior majoring in sociology and elementary education. As time went on, we started to talk across the aisle, and as we came closer to Philadelphia, I realized that I wanted to see this gorgeous girl again. I also tell the story sometimes, but it is factually not true, that on this flight I noticed Linda's mother before I saw her. And I said to myself, "What a great looking mother, I wish she had a daughter. I would like to meet her."

We talked about my work, and I gave Linda my business card, asking her to give me a call when she was in Philadelphia. It was my psychiatrist business card. Linda must have wondered whether I thought she needed to see a psychiatrist. I had been married to Crista almost ten years and was clearly not experienced in dating in America. After a while, Linda asked me whether I would like to have her telephone number, and I said yes. She wrote it on a napkin for me. By the time we landed in Philadelphia, Linda's father had Larry on his lap looking out of the window.

You must understand that I was rather nervous about all this for many reasons. In addition to being a recent widower and having no experience dating, I was much older than Linda, and had a son. Well, after several days I found the courage to call Linda and set up a date. I took her to the Kona Kai at the Marriott on City Line Avenue. We enjoyed ourselves tremendously and decided to meet again. The third date was at Café Careme at the former Philadelphia Sheraton, at that time one of the best restaurants in the city. I wanted to impress her and ordered caviar, which is very salty. But she had just had her wisdom teeth removed that afternoon. The caviar was too salty for the still healing wound in her mouth, and she could not eat it. Linda never tried caviar again, which saved me a lot of money over the years.

On our last date before Linda had to return to Salem College for her senior year, Linda, Larry and I went to the Schwenksville Folk Festival. We sat on the ground on a blanket and listened to James Taylor. Even when I first met Linda, I could tell she loved Larry. As our relationship developed, I knew she would raise him as if he were her own son.

Early in my relationship with Linda, I constantly and compulsively showed her the slides and films of my trips with Larry and Crista. Linda was so understanding; she must have perceived that I was working through my grief. Even as a young woman, she was so warm and compassionate.

Soon thereafter, Linda went back to school, where she decided to add German to her language studies. Linda had studied German for only one year, but by the time of our honeymoon she spoke it almost fluently. While dating Linda, I visited Winston-Salem several times and I met most of her close friends. Larry came with me once or twice. Over Christmas we went skiing at Camelback Mountain Resort in the Pocono Mountains. After only one hour of lessons, showing very poor judgment, I took Linda to the top of the mountain. Poor Linda had to get down the hill traversing and sidestepping—that was all she had been taught in her one lesson.

Just imagine how scared and angry she must have been. Linda let me know about it, quite rightfully so. This was the first and last skiing Linda did with me for quite some time.

Courtship and Marriage

Our courtship was short and swift; we got engaged at Christmas. As a well-brought-up young man, I requested an audition with Linda's father and asked him for permission to marry his daughter. This is a tradition I'm proud to say my boys followed when they planned to get married. Only many years later, after Linda had passed away, did I come across a stack of letters from our courtship that contained a letter I had forgotten about. I had written this letter to Linda's mother in late November 1963 requesting her support for my courtship. This letter was saved all these years, first by Linda's mother and later by Linda. It speaks for itself and my concern at that time. It is attached in the Appendix. I learned later that Linda's mother, whom my grandchildren later called "Nana Bee," had also lost her mother when she was eight years old. And Grandma Tyler, Nana Bee's stepmother, raised her. Because of her similar personal experience, Grandma Tyler always supported my courtship with Linda.

Linda's father had some reservations, though. He was initially worried that I might not be able to keep up with raising young children due to my age. I can't say that I blame him. Luckily for my children and me, age never was a problem, and my younger boys, Mike and Steve, never looked at me as an old man. Having turned 86 recently, I am finally starting to realize that I am not sixty years old anymore. I find myself hesitating whether or not I shall ski one more year—at least not the black diamond runs. My age did not keep me, however, from playing two days of soccer in a tournament at Eagles Mere with my grandchildren and some fathers this past summer. It was a special tournament that Andrew and Peter signed me and their father up for. How could I turn this invitation down?

During our courtship, I learned that Linda's father was secretary-treasurer and vice president of Sun Oil and was on the board of directors. Linda lived with her family in Pitman, New Jersey. Pitman was a town of nine thousand residents. On July 4, 2008, I saw a large newspaper article about the Fourth of July parade held there each year. It reminded me of how lovely Linda's childhood must have been. Her grandparents on her father's side also lived in Pitman. Her grandfather worked for IBM for many years and when I met him he was still on its board of directors. He was living on his one-hundred-acre nursery farm in Pitman. He was a tall, impressive, wonderful person, as was his wife, Linda's grandmother. We visited them on their farm many times until both departed from this earth much too early. They had loaned us the funds to buy the property behind our house on Sweetbriar Road, and over several Christmas holidays forgave us the loan as a gift. I also have several South American-themed oil paintings that we received from them as gifts. They are still my favorite paintings.

While Linda's father's background was in New Jersey and Pennsylvania with a college and masters degree in accounting, Linda's mother, "Bee," grew up in Boston. Her ancestry goes all the way back to William Bradford, who came from England to America on the Mayflower in 1620. Bee belonged to the Descendents of the Mayflower and also to The Colonial Dames of America. I certainly did not realize when I dated Linda what a famous ancestor she had. Growing up, Bee spent the summer months at their cottage on Cape Cod in Dennis near Hyannis Port. She was an avid sailor.

After she completed college she was one of the first twenty young women hired by IBM to be trained for junior leadership positions, a first in America at that time.

Our wedding was held on June 27, 1964, at the Episcopal church of Pitman in ninety-five degree heat. My friend, John Morris, was my best man, and my friend, Mickey Stunkard, chair of the Department of Psychiatry at Penn at that time, was in the wedding party, together with Linda's brothers: Chuck, Jack, and Jim. My sister, Gisela, came from Germany, and naturally Larry and Crista's mother, Ellie, were also at the wedding. The reception was held on Linda's grandparents' estate, the receiving line was in an English garden, and the festivities were held under a big tent on the lawn next to the lake. The women were beautiful, and the men wore white tuxedos. It was gorgeous.

My parents could not come, as my father did not fly. I have also wondered if he felt uncomfortable attending because he was embarrassed that he lost his earlier business and went through bankruptcy.

On our honeymoon we visited the World's Fair in New York and then boarded the SS Leonardo da Vinci, crossing the Atlantic from New York to Cannes, France. We took our white Thunderbird with us. The Atlantic crossing was wonderful. The weather was great, but what was even more enjoyable was meeting a young Texan couple. They had traveled to Europe on the ship before, so they brought together about eight young couples from among the passengers, and we became friends. Each couple would throw a cocktail party before dinner, and we did many things together.

At Cannes, Linda and I and our car were unloaded and we stayed for several days at the Carlton Hotel, with a room overlooking the sea. We caught up with our Texan friends at Villa D'Este on Lake Como after a nice Italian man fixed my flat tire earlier that day.

I vividly remember the dancing under the stars on the terrace after dinner. But I also remember that the milk we got for breakfast was warm and curdled. I used a linen table napkin as a sieve and thus was able to provide Linda with unclotted milk for her coffee. At that time, even the famous Vila D'Este was not yet air-conditioned. From there we traveled to St. Moritz, where we stayed at the Palace Hotel. On our trip to Vienna from St. Moritz, we stayed overnight at the hotel on the Gross-Glockner Pass, one of the highest in the Alps overlooking the glacier. From Vienna we traveled to Salzburg, and we stayed in Schloss Fuschel, where Linda encouraged me to ride on a horse with her, which I, like a loving puppy, gladly did.

We visited many other places, such as Munich, Hamburg, Bremen, and Langeoog, an island in the North Sea. We also visited Berlin and crossed to East Berlin via Checkpoint Charley. We returned to Frankfurt via Muenster, my university town and visited Gisela and her family, as well as Willich and Krefeld, where my parents lived at that time. We also drove the Romantic Road and stayed overnight in the Eisenhuth, one of the most romantic hotels in Rothenburg ob der Tauber, a very old town that was only marginally damaged during World War II.

At the end of our European trip we picked Larry up at a beach near Knokke, Holland, where he had been camping with Crista's family. We left the next day to board the ferry to England, and then drove our car on the carriageway to London, where we arrived late at night. To help you picture this seemingly mundane thing, keep in mind I was driving an American car in England, sitting in the left-hand seat and driving on the left side of the road. We stayed at the Grosvenor House Hotel—the very same hotel Linda had stayed in with her parents on her trip the year before. One night we went to Roules for dinner. She had remembered it as the restaurant where she enjoyed "such a great rose wine." We found out it was a Mateus Rose.

After a few days in London, we drove to Birmingham for the 1964 CINP meeting. When we arrived, we were surprised to discover that all of the Americans in attendance—not that there were many—were staying in university dormitories. This was quite a change from a five-star hotel that we'd had at previous meetings, and not what this honeymoon couple had expected. We didn't stay long. A few days later we drove back to London and prepared to return to Philadelphia, while our car was shipped to New York.

We were heading home. This was a pattern we would repeat many times in the coming years.

It was always good to head home.

Again, as so often happened in my life, serendipity, or perhaps an angel, must have watched over Larry and me. How else could it happen that not long after Crista's death, Larry found a second mother who loved him and would raise him and I found my second wife?

5

The Era of Psychopharmacology

With a new wife and a new life ahead of me, I was excited about what the future might hold. I returned to my field of study with great enthusiasm, amidst great change in the young field of psychopharmacology.

After 1962, when the Kefauver Harris Amendment to the Food, Drug, and Cosmetic Act became law, the Food and Drug Administration (FDA) also had to consider efficacy when approving new medications. The amendment was written by public officials and lawyers, and says nothing about methodology. It was left up to the scientists to develop appropriate methodology.

Before 1962, only safety had to be assessed by the FDA, and this only after rather cursory review. Thus there was no incentive for the industry to carry out placebo or drug-controlled, double-blind clinical trials. All drugs introduced into psychiatry in the 1950s and early 1960s were studied mainly in open trials, often with only global outcome assessment. It took many years before these newly-introduced drugs into psychiatry were subjected to rigorous, placebo-controlled trials.

Trial methodology in the '60s was in its infancy. The only controlled research was conducted by the Veteran's Administration and by a few NIMH-supported centers. The 1962 amendment, however, did not inform the FDA how to define efficacy. It only provided strong impetus to develop better clinical research methodology. It took the FDA until the late 1970s to develop and publish guidelines for the evaluation of various psychiatric drugs. This was done with the help of a young elite organization called the American College of Neuro-Psychopharmacology (ACNP), of which I was a charter member, and another group of researchers who were part of the Early Clinical Drug Evaluation Unit (ECDEU) of the Psychopharmacology Research Branch of NIMH, of which I was also an early member. Dr. Wittenborn was the chair of the guideline development project. Our research area was defined as neurotic anxiety, and I thus had the fortune of being part of this process of developing drug evaluation guidelines for the FDA.

The new amendment to the FDA law led to the establishment of the Drug Efficacy Study of the National Academy of Sciences, whose goal it was to review all drugs approved for marketing by the FDA between 1938 and 1962. This process lasted from about 1965 to 1967. Drugs marketed before 1938 were grandfathered and could stay on the market. The result of this study led to a large reduction of drugs previously approved by the FDA. I had the good fortune of being a member of the panel responsible for psychiatric drugs. The panel was under the leadership of Dr. Danny Freedman, chair of psychiatry at the University of Chicago and later editor of the premier psychiatric journal, *Archives of General Psychiatry.* One benefit this free public service provided was that one of the meetings was held in New Orleans during Mardi Gras, which the committee members attended together with their wives. Of sixty-five drugs reviewed, thirty-one were found to be inactive and were later removed from the market.

Some years later, in 1972, I was asked by the FDA to chair an advisory review panel on Over-the-Counter (OTC) Daytime and Nighttime Sedative and Stimulant products, which conducted its review from 1972 to 1975. This review led to the elimination or reformulation of many OTC medications marketed at that time. The results of a study conducted by our group, published in the *Journal of the American Medical Association,* contributed significantly to this review. Among other things, the study clearly showed that the highly advertised OTC daytime sedative, Compoz, was completely void of any anxiolytic properties.

One of the first publications presenting state-of-the-art, research methodology in the late 1960s was a book entitled *Principles and Problems in Establishing the Efficacy of Psychotropic Agents.* I was editor of the methodology section in this book and contributor of two chapters. This was followed with the publication of FDA guidelines for the evaluation of psychiatric drugs in 1978, another effort in which I was heavily involved, and was revisited in 1994 with the book, *Clinical Evaluation of Psychotropic Drugs,* and for which I was one of the four section editors. Both publications were conducted under the sponsorship of the NIMH and ACNP. Clearly, research methodology was advanced by academia, not industry.

A New Science

The mid- to late-1950s and early 1960s were exciting years. A new science was born, and, for the first time, pharmacological tools became available to significantly help mankind. And I was directly in the middle of it! I soon became one of the leading international experts in the assessment and pharmacological treatment of anxiety neurosis. Many of the drugs marketed in the 1950s and early 1960s for the treatment of anxiety did not live up to their initial promise, however, and eventually only a few were found to be more effective and safer than the barbiturates. With time, meprobamate (Miltown) was replaced by newer anti-anxiety drugs called, because of their chemical structure, benzodiazepines. Drugs such as Librium and Valium (sometimes referred to as "mother's little helper") became household words. These two drugs were later followed by others of the same class, such as Ativan, Xanax and Klonopin.

Introduced in 1963, Valium was, by the late 1960s, the most frequently prescribed medication in the world. In one study Librium was used to tranquilize lions and tigers in the San Diego Zoo. This was followed by newspaper headlines that read, "The drug that tames wild tigers … what will it do for nervous women?" The benzodiazepines were enthusiastically accepted in the '60s and '70s, only to be attacked soon thereafter, mostly by British psychiatrists. For example, in 1978 one British psychiatrist called them the "opium of the masses."

In America, Barbara Gordon wrote the book, *I'm Dancing as Fast as I Can.* In it, the author described a horrible experience with Valium "addiction" and her attempts to stop taking Valium. My interpretation of her story was that the author was suffering from a severe borderline personality disorder and should never have been placed on Valium in the first place. And, in fact, she later did quite well when treated with a neuroleptic (antipsychotic) medication. Some puritans in our society expressed belief that anything that is prescribed this much must be bad. This is a belief I never shared. If a person was doing well with a crutch, such as having a Valium pill in a pocket for emergency use, was that so terrible? It was fine with me. Valium was certainly being taken for all kinds of little ills. And this was during a time when everyone believed anxiety was only short-lived. These new drugs were also excellent "as needed" medications, since they worked almost immediately. I was one of only a few academics who suggested that, like diabetes, anxiety for some patients could be a chronic disorder, and that long-term use of benzodiazepines might be appropriate. Had we known as much about anxiety at that time as we do now, much of what was termed over-treatment or prolonged treatment would today be considered appropriate treatment. Many of the patients who were described as being hooked on therapeutic doses of benzodiazepines might, in fact, only have been in need of long-term treatment for their anxiety disorder.

And while, indeed, the benzodiazepines such as Valium caused low-dose physical dependence in some patients when used for several months, antidepressants, which today have largely replaced the benzodiazepines in the treatment of anxiety by psychiatrists, also cause discontinuation symptoms, have many gastrointestinal (GI) and sexual adverse effects, and their onset of beneficial effects takes several weeks. In my treatment of anxiety disorders with benzodiazepines, I have yet to encounter a private patient I couldn't safely discontinue from his benzodiazepine use, if I considered it appropriate. It is most interesting that even today more prescriptions per year are written for benzodiazepines than for antidepressants for anxious patients in family practice.

In July 2008, I chaired a symposium at the CINP congress in Munich discussing the role of the benzodiazepines in the twenty-first century. Hundreds of psychiatrists and other mental health workers filled the large ballroom. The conclusion of our symposium discussions was that the benzodiazepines today are probably not over-prescribed, but under-prescribed. They are clearly clinically effective and safe medications, if appropriately used, and so far, no better medication has been found to replace them.

While working at Penn in the late 1950s and early 1960s, I learned how hard it was to persuade psychoanalysts that medications had a place in psychiatry. Psychoanalysts occupied most chairs of psychiatric academic centers. Most held an attitude that drugs interfered with psychotherapy and should not be used, not even with schizophrenia. It was their belief that patients had to continue to experience anxiety and depression in order to benefit from psychoanalysis. The treatment offered by many psychiatrists at that time, in my opinion, bordered on malpractice. It took more than a decade until medication was hesitatingly accepted by academia as appropriate treatment for schizophrenic patients. It took even longer to integrate antidepressant treatment and anxiolytic treatment into outpatient therapy.

Even in the early 1970s, the view of anxiety was not much different. Anxiety was still treated with psychotherapy, or very often the anxiety was unrecognized and not treated at all. Anti-anxiety medications were to be prescribed only rarely, as most anxieties were considered short-lived and not *true* psychiatric illnesses. Yet non-psychiatrists learned very early that many of their patients suffered from chronic anxiety, resulting in severe disabilities, and requiring treatment for longer periods of time. At that time some physicians were blamed for addicting patients to benzodiazepines. In fact, a few leading experts called the use of benzodiazepines inappropriate. This made many of us wonder whether the resistance to the use of medication by many psychiatrists was possibly motivated by monetary factors.

In private psychiatric hospitals, psychoanalysis continued to be used as the only treatment, even for psychotic or depressed patients, and the newer medications were rejected. At that time one had to be poor to receive the right treatment, meaning medication instead of psychoanalysis. Psychoanalysis was the treatment for the rich, for the patients who could afford it. Resistance in analysis might draw out treatment for months or years, which provided bread and butter for the analyst who only needed fewer than ten patients to provide all his income. Therefore, psychopharmacology encountered strong resistance from the psychiatric establishment.

In the treatment of depression, the drugs of choice were the tricyclics, and particularly imipramine (Tofranil) and amitriptyline (Elavil). The MAO inhibitors, such as phenelzine (Nardil), while clearly effective, have never become frequently-used drugs in the US because patients had to keep a tyramine-free diet, which was quite difficult. For example, patients could not drink red wine or eat cheese, to mention only two of the dietary restrictions.

At the same time, in the excitement about this new therapy, clinical results produced by psychopharmacology often were overenthusiastically interpreted and may have promised too much. Instead of introducing the new drugs as a way of helping patients address and deal with their problems, many physicians promised prescriptions of these new drugs as a panacea to solve all of the patients' problems.

Despite all these obstacles, it was a time of great discovery. One became an expert by doing and experimenting, not by learning from one's elders. There *were* no elders in this new therapeutic field. From the beginning, I was interested in the outpatient treatment of anxious and depressed patients, this during a time when psychiatrists in training who entered the field of psychopharmacology focused primarily on inpatient psychiatry, while most others stayed away from psychopharmacology all together, following the holy grail of psychoanalysis.

Adding to Our Family

It was during this time of great discovery in my field that Linda and I began to think of adding to our family. Regretfully, despite our attempts to have a baby for several years, including infertility treatments, we were still unsuccessful in 1971. And then suddenly, providence contributed to our family's growth.

In the spring of 1971, my father suffered a stroke that affected mainly his speech center. I flew to Frankfurt in early summer and visited with him for about a week. During my visit, I went one day to play golf at the Kronberg golf course, where I was paired up with another man for our round of golf.

I learned that he was Father Beck, a married Catholic priest. Father Beck had converted to the Catholic faith after serving as a married Lutheran priest. A special dispensation allowed him to become the priest at a Roman Catholic Church in the Frankfurt area that served the families of the American armed forces. During our round of golf, he shared with me that one of his main interests was to counsel and help pregnant women who could not keep their children, once born, if they wanted to preserve their marriages. Abortion was no option for a Catholic, only adoption.

By that time, we still had several holes of golf to play. I poured out my heart to him that my young wife, Linda, and I had been trying for several years to have a baby, and we would love to adopt a child if the chance existed.

"Well," Father Beck responded, "I am counseling just now a twenty-year-old girl whose husband had been out of the country as part of his army duty, and while he was gone the poor girl became involved with a German graduate student and is now pregnant."

The husband was willing to forgive his wife for her indiscretion, but was not able to raise the child as his own. Husband and wife were eager to place the baby with a loving family who would raise the child in the Catholic faith.

You can imagine how thrilled I was. As soon as I got back to the house of my sister, Gisela, I telephoned Linda. She was so excited that she wanted to come to Frankfurt at once. The next day, I visited Father Beck in his parish home, and Gisela, and her husband, Ahmad, had him over to their home soon thereafter.

The baby, we did not know whether boy or girl, was expected in late September or early October. I planned to fly home right away and set everything in motion on our end. Then Linda and I would return to Frankfurt long before the baby's delivery date to visit with Father Beck together and make the final adoption arrangements.

Suddenly, however, my father passed away, bringing Linda and me to Frankfurt even sooner than planned to attend my father's funeral. And, so it happened, as the Lord takes away the Lord also gives. We knew that not long after my father left this earth, our new baby would enter and be part of our family.

After some time, and once all of the paperwork was completed, my work forced me to return to Gladwyne earlier than planned, leaving Linda with Gisela and Ahmad, waiting for the arrival of our new baby. Our son, Stephen, was born on October 3, 1971. Father Beck took Linda to the US Army hospital where Steve's birth mother handed him over to Linda. The next day Steve was baptized by Father Beck at my sister's home. And a few days later Linda, with Steve in her arms, arrived at Philadelphia International Airport.

In the meantime, I had everything ready for our baby's arrival, though I must admit that Linda had the baby's room prepared long before we both flew to Frankfurt in late summer.

Steve was barely with us for six months when after so many years of trying, Linda became pregnant with our second son, Michael. So we joined the Catholic church in Gladwyne and raised both boys Roman Catholic. Father O'Halloran, our Gladwyne priest, was a wonderful person. He included Linda in all parish activities, knowing full well that she was not a Catholic, but an Episcopalian. Suddenly, as Larry was close to college age, we had the pleasure of raising two baby boys, Steve and Mike, who were just one-and-a-half years apart in age. Our lives were fulfilled.

Research and Discovery

As of this writing, I have just completed the last year of a six-year multimillion-dollar NIMH grant studying long-term medication treatment in anxiety disorders. When I submitted this grant almost eight years ago, many friends and colleagues asked why I was still submitting grant applications at my age. Here is the reason. The young, aspiring psychiatric researchers whom I was training gave me all kinds of excuses why they were unable to attract NIMH grants. When I told them about my success with grants, they complained that it was easy years ago, but not today. And so I had to show these young psychiatrists that the old man was still able to obtain federal grant support. And I did.

During this process, Linda was worried that I would be disappointed if I didn't get my grant. Yet this thought never crossed my mind. I was convinced of the importance of my proposed research, and thus worked harder on each resubmission until I finally was successful, much to Linda's relief.

When asked why I am still working at my advanced age, my usual response is, "But I am not working, I am having fun." Every day I look forward to my work, which involves research, patient care, teaching, and administration. And it was good that I liked my work, because Linda always told me, "I married you for better and for worse, but not for lunch." Linda always supported this workaholic!

Had Dr. Appel not given me the chance to enter psychopharmacology, I don't know where in psychiatry I would have ended up. Luckily for me, Dr. Appel guided me well.

I recently reviewed my late 1950s and early 1960s tax returns. I earned very little money at the university during that time and actually brought in more than my university salary from outside work, mainly from private clinical practice, but also from consulting with research departments of various pharmaceutical companies. I never consulted for marketing, and I never belonged to an industry speakers bureau. I was involved in interpreting animal results and developing clinical trial protocols for potential anti-anxiety and antidepressant experimental medications.

I also had become the consulting psychiatrist for the German Consulate General in Philadelphia, evaluating Jewish patients who were persecuted by the Nazis and had rightful claims for pension from the German government. I saw many hundreds of formerly persecuted patients, many of them at that time living in Vineland and working as chicken farmers. Subjecting a variety of data—such as persecution history, anxiety, depression, and many other factors—collected in several hundred patients to a multivariate analysis to search for predictors of present degree of psychopathology (now called post-traumatic stress disorder or PTSD), we found that the strongest predictor was not time nor severity of persecution, but survivor guilt of those who left alive extermination camps such as

Auschwitz. My son, Larry, helped with the analysis of this data as a senior special project while at Penn. I had a part-time German secretary at that time, as I had to complete all my reports in German.

Reviewing my early presentations at the CINP, at that time the only scientific group that brought all people interested in the new field of psychopharmacology together, I was one of the few reporting on methodology, placebo response, and the effect that nonspecific factors had on drug response in anxiety and depression. In my early publications, I stressed the fact that drugs were there to facilitate psychotherapy, not given out of a black box without patient-therapist interactions.

It is most regrettable today that insurance companies want to divorce drugs from psychotherapy treatment. How can a psychiatrist treat a patient appropriately with medication within a twenty-minute time limit? It still is true, even today, that drugs are most effective if prescribed by a caring physician who understands that psychiatric medications are not a panacea to solve all the patient's problems, but rather tools to help the patients begin to work on solving their issues. Clearly, drugs are not effective if prescribed in lieu of empathy and caring.

Homebody

Considering my heavy involvement in the new science of psychopharmacology, one may ask why I never was an elected officer in one of these organizations, or why I never became a chairman of psychiatry at a university. I thought about this question a great deal. One obvious possibility is that I might not make a good chairman, or was not qualified enough, yet I had several offers from American psychiatry departments, and even one from a leading German university. I also had an offer from a large international pharmaceutical company to become its senior vice-president of its central nervous system (CNS) division. But I always chose to stay at Penn. Penn has always been good to me; and bringing in large sums of research funds to Penn every year gave me the independence I treasured.

There was, however, a time or two when I got restless. After one of these times, the university offered me an endowed chair, the Stuart and Emily Mudd Professor of Human Behavior Chair, to expand my research activities into OB-GYN. For several years until its closure, I also was chair of psychiatry at the Philadelphia General Hospital, which in the 1960s and 1970s was one of the leading public city teaching hospitals in the country. And for one year I was asked to be chief of the Philadelphia Marriage Council to save the institution from financial disaster.

One reason for my not assuming national or international administrative and elected positions is probably a psychological one. While in some ways I am rather outgoing, in other ways I am not. I liked my science and my national and international reputation. I enjoyed flying all over the world as the leading psychiatrist in my area of expertise. I flew on the supersonic Concorde at least ten times. The fact that in America you are known by your accomplishments, and not by your academic title, also played a part. This is quite different in Germany, where you have to be a chair of a department to be recognized. It took me many years to build up my Private Practice Research Group for conducting clinical trial research outside the ivy walls of academia. It was the only group of its kind in the world at that time, and it would have been next to impossible to build such a group while serving as a department chairman. Thus, despite offers from institutions in both Germany and America, I decided to stay at Penn.

But to a large extent, these might all be rationalizations. To be honest, I had immigrated once; I didn't want to move again. In many ways I was, and still am, a homebody who likes to spend as much time as possible at home with his family. After the children were in bed, I could still do some work if I had too. And finally, the Philadelphia and Main Line area was a wonderful place to raise a family. Linda and I were happy where we lived. And though we moved twice after we were married, both moves were within a mile from each other and both were in Gladwyne. We lived for 21 years at Sweetbriar Road and since 1986 in our present house on Youngsford Road.

Linda and I tried to attend as many of our children's interscholastic activities as possible, and believe me there were many, which meant that I frequently had to leave work at two thirty in the afternoon, and would try to catch up with my work in the evening after dinner.

As a family we spent our vacations together at the shore in our Avalon, New Jersey, beach house. Steve and Mike sailed Sunfish boats and won many tournaments, despite the fact that they only spent half the summer sailing. Some of our friends, whose children dedicated the whole summer to sailing Sunfish, would be upset when their children lost out in the trophies to our sons. Almost every summer, I wrote NIMH research grant applications while vacationing in Avalon. Computers were not yet available, so I wrote them by hand and used a Dictaphone. My secretary would come out once a week for a beach day and pick up my material for transcribing via her typewriter in the office.

We also took skiing vacations each Christmas and Presidents Day weekend at our ski-in, ski-out condo in Stowe, Vermont, and in the Rockies over spring vacation or, when the boys were in college, over the New Year's holiday. We also frequently went to Europe, combining vacations with scientific meetings or consulting activity. Once the boys were out of college, Linda and I often traveled alone, as our travel calendar didn't fit with those of young men in new jobs and with young families.

I must mention here one particular time in Berlin, when close friends of ours invited us for dinner. It was during the World Congress of Biological Psychiatry in 2001. For many years I had been a consultant to two leading German pharmaceutical companies and had helped them to develop a few, rather successful, compounds. This dinner was arranged and planned for one of these companies by our friend. Since our friend was also a business associate, we expected a nice restaurant, but what a surprise when we arrived at the venue of the dinner. It was the Casino on the Wannsee in West Berlin, next to a fancy restaurant at the Glienicker Bruecke, a former crossing point from West-Berlin into the Russian East Zone of Germany.

The Casino was a small summer palace of the Prussian kings and is now a museum. We were taken into a large dining room with windows overlooking the Wannsee and a view of the setting sun. The Michelin star chef running the nearby restaurant for this evening was our personal chef. For that evening, he was there only for us, and particularly for Linda and me, the guests of honor. It was a gorgeous evening with the most delicious food. Can you imagine how surprised and honored we were when we were told that the Casino had been opened for dinner only *four times* to entertain foreign guests since the end of World War II. Besides Linda and me, the other guests were Bill Clinton, Tony Blair, and Francois Mitterand.

In June 2009, I took my son Steve, and his wife, Heidi, along with their fifteen-month-old son, Aiden, to visit my sister, Gisela, and her family, which included five children and nineteen grandchildren in Eschborn near Frankfurt. After visiting family we traveled by train to Berlin to show my children where I grew up. One evening Heidi and Steve visited one of Heidi's college friends who had married a German and had just been transferred to Berlin. So I invited my old friends to dinner at Hugos, a famous restaurant at the InterContinental Berlin—the same hotel where Linda and I had stayed on our honeymoon. Hugos is run by a chef with a Michelin star who prepared a special eight-course dinner for us. This was our way of saying thank you to our Berlin friends for their previous kindness.

I have been very lucky in my professional life. Many of my business associates and colleagues became good friends, and our contact continued long after our professional liaison had terminated. I readily admit that my selection of research collaborators was always somewhat biased. I never worked with anyone whom I did not like or did not trust. I turned down millions of dollars in research grants because I did not like the people or the sponsor with whom I would have had to work.

Serendipity may have provided me with lots of opportunities in life, but it was still up to me to decide which paths to take. I took the ones that were more about people, family, and patients, not money. This is a lesson that has served me well.

6

Three Influential Organizations

I do not know who invented the name of psychopharmacology, but it must have been coined somewhere around the time of the discovery of chlorpromazine (Thorazine) in France in 1952. Since computers, faxes, the Internet, and even Federal Express didn't exist at that time, the distribution of new findings took a rather circuitous route. It was usually fastest when presented at a swiftly-arranged symposium, separate from any established organization. International travel was very expensive at the time, and only hardy souls would travel to Europe by either ship or a propeller air plane for a short meeting. Consequently, at the first few meetings in Europe, with the focus on this new tranquilizer, only very few American clinicians and scientists were present.

Given the negative environment towards the use of drugs in psychiatry, it is understandable that those interested in this new field founded groups that included all disciplines interested in psychiatric drug development. I had the great opportunity to be involved as a young man in the founding of the three leading organizations in Psychopharmacology, which were all started about fifty years ago. The first small symposium, which was arranged to discuss Thorazine, was held in Paris in October 1955. Thorazine was the first drug discovered to treat schizophrenic symptoms, and thus the first modern psychiatric drug. It speaks to the clinical and observational astuteness of the early clinicians that these open-label findings held up to later scrutiny. The first American publication on chlorpromazine, which appeared about that time was almost fully rejected by the psychoanalytic establishment that controlled American psychiatry.

Collegium Internationale Neuro-Psychopharmacologicum (CINP)

The next symposium focusing on antipsychotic medications was held in Milan in May 1957. Again, pharmacologists, not clinicians, sponsored it. Here, for the first time, a few participants talked about starting a new scientific organization to bring scientists from many different fields and from all over the world together. But further discussion was postponed until the second World Congress of Psychiatry, which was held in Zurich in September 1957. That year the CINP was founded when a Basel-based pharmacologist named Rothlin called a small group of people together for dinner at the train station in Zurich and presented the invitees with a slate of officers that included him as president. Thus, the first international psychopharmacological organization began without any discussion and without any confirmatory vote.

In later years, several pharmacologists and psychiatrists were honored with the Lasker Award, a prestigious award given for major contributions to medical science. Laborit and Deniker from France received the award for their work on Thorazine, Lehmann from Canada for his work with imipramine, and Nathan Kline was honored for his work with reserpine, the main ingredient of the snakeroot rauwolfia serpentina, an old Indian remedy. Kline is the only psychiatrist to receive two Lasker Awards; the second for his discovery that the antituberculosis drug, Marsilid, had antidepressant properties. None of these revolutionaries was a chair in academic centers, or even a full-time academic, and I don't believe any of them had ever conducted a placebo-controlled clinical trial. All were astute clinicians and observers and believers in the new psychiatric treatment with medications.

The CINP had its first of many congresses in Rome in 1958, and it was there that the CINP was officially founded. I attended that meeting and became one of the group's first members. Though it started unofficially with thirty-two members at the Zurich train station, there were sixty-five members from all over the world when it was established officially. Focus at the first several CINP congresses was almost exclusively on Thorazine and Serpasil and on psychedelic substances such as LSD and Mescaline, studied primarily as facilitators of psychotherapy and as tools to study other drugs. Stimulants and drugs such as morphine and barbiturates had a much higher place in the interest of the congress than anti-anxiety drugs such as meprobamate. In fact, meprobamate was hardly mentioned. At the Rome meeting I presented a paper on the methodology of drug evaluation in neurotic outpatients, and at the second congress in Basel, in 1960, I presented a paper discussing results obtained with the cold pressure test in drug evaluation.

One particular incident still stands out in my mind. During the election of officers at the 1960 Basel annual meeting, two US groups were fighting each other furiously. I sat in the audience with some German colleagues who couldn't believe what was going on. They told me that if this happened between two German groups, they would become lifelong enemies. I responded, "Wait until after the meeting." As I had suspected, after the meeting both US groups had met for cocktails at the bar, congratulating each other on their exchange of ideas. This is an excellent example of why I emigrated to America and became a US citizen: the freedom of speech and the ability to separate professional disagreements from personal interactions.

The third congress was held in Munich in 1962, and I presented two papers dealing with the placebo response. Crista was with me at that time, already aware of her ovarian cancer. At the same time, my colleague, Seymour Fisher, from the NIMH, presented some of our early data collected in the first ever collaborative outpatient trial with anxious patients. The study was a collaborative effort between NIMH, Johns Hopkins Medical School, and the University of Pennsylvania.

All my presentations at these early CINP congresses dealt with the methodology of placebo-controlled drug evaluations, with particular focus on the role of nonspecific factors on treatment response. This early interest of mine in the treatment of anxious and depressed neurotic outpatients was also evident at the fourth CINP congress held in Birmingham, England, in 1964, where I was a discussant at the symposium, "Dynamics and Significance of Psychopharmacologic Interventions in Psychiatry."

This meeting was held at the end of our honeymoon, after Linda and I had enjoyed a six-week trip through Western Europe. We had our white Thunderbird with us, and I can vividly remember driving one hundred miles per hour on the freeway between London to Birmingham, yet still being passed by many British cars, primarily Jaguars. From then on, Linda accompanied me to most international meetings. The next CINP meeting was held in Washington, DC in 1966, and Linda, the young bride, was the star of the show. The attendance in these early meetings was small. Everyone knew each other, and many of us either were already friends or soon became friends.

When I attended the 1970 CINP meeting, my father and mother drove with Linda and me in a rented car from Frankfurt to Prague. On the way we visited several enormous castles in southern Germany. We then spent a few days in Marienbad, where Linda and I played golf. We were still behind the Iron Curtain at that time. From there we also visited Karlsbad. This was the last time that my father came on a trip with us. He died the next year, in 1971. The 1970 congress was the first time that I presented our revolutionary concept of carrying out clinical trials in family practice, instead of in academic centers and large hospital clinics. It was at the Quebec meeting in 1976 when I shifted my research focus away from the beneficial effects of the benzodiazepines to their potential limitations.

Over the years, our children (and sometimes, my mother) often accompanied Linda and me to the CINP and World Congresses. But, in the early '70s, one did not travel with small children. Linda stayed home, and I either traveled alone or with Larry or my mother, or both together. For example, my mother joined me at the congress in Vienna in 1978, and to her delight, we stayed at the fanciest hotel in Vienna, the Hotel Imperial. In 1980, for the Goeteburg CINP congress, Linda decided Steve and Mike were old enough to travel overseas. We flew with them to Frankfurt, and went alone to Goeteburg while my mother flew with the boys to Oslo, where we later met to visit Norway and Sweden together. We took the train from Oslo over the snowy mountains to Bergen, and from there flew to Stockholm.

In 1982 all three boys came with us to London. We then visited Cairo and the pharaoh's burial grounds at Luxor, and then went on to Rome, Athens, and Frankfurt. A visit to Frankfurt, and the home of my sister, Gisela, and her husband, Ahmad, was a *must* on most of our trips. And they do not even live in Frankfurt, but in the western suburb of Eschborn. Aunt Gisela and Uncle Ahmad were my sons' favorite aunt and uncle, and the same is true for my grandchildren. Ahmad taught my sons, and my two older grandsons, the higher levels of chess and backgammon. And "Frankfurt" also included my parents when they were still alive. They had an apartment in my sister's house.

In 1984, my mother joined me in Florence and Venice. The meeting was during school time and Linda could not come with the younger boys. At another meeting in Europe, Larry and I skied in Zuers, Austria. It was at that time that Larry studied for a year in Vienna. In 1984 we again went to Europe for one of our niece's wedding. Before the wedding, we visited another cousin in Munich, and visited Garmish-Partenkirchen, located at the foot of the Zugspitze, the highest mountain in Germany.

We combined the 1988 CINP congress with a car trip through Bavaria and Austria before we ended up in Munich. This was the year that Steve and Mike discovered that the Frankfurt McDonald's served beer without an age limit. On the trip through Austria, the van, which Steve was driving, lost its clutch. We called the Austrian AAA, and while we waited at an empty, but friendly, restaurant for a few hours in the afternoon, the AAA delivered us two cars, as they didn't have a van big enough for all our luggage and us. So, despite a severe backache, I also had to drive. We spent a few days at a famous Bavarian Lake, the Herrenchiemsee, where I stayed mostly in the hotel bed pumped full of codeine. In a few days, however, I was much better, and we drove to Munich, where Linda and I stayed for the CINP meeting, and my mother took Steve and Mike back to her home in Frankfurt, where we picked them up a few days later. At the Munich congress in 1988, I organized and co-chaired with Otto Benkert, MD, from Mainz University, the symposium, "Methodology of the Evaluation of Psychotropic Drugs," the content of which was later published in a book of the same title, often cited and referred to by researchers in the field.

Until about 1978, all CINP presentations were published in the proceedings, volumes entitled *Neuro-Psychopharmacology,* but as the CINP grew, this was not possible any more. Symposia and other activities were frequently published separately or not at all.

The CINP congresses were always an important venue for me to exchange ideas with leaders in the field from all over the world, but particularly with my many friends from North America, England and the German-speaking countries, many of whom were psychiatry department chairmen at that time. For example, in 1992, in Nice, I chaired a benzodiazepine symposium. Linda, our friends, the Freemans, and I traveled together through France prior to arriving in Nice.

In 1996, the congress was in Melbourne, Australia, and Steve came with me. Linda was chair of an important cancer charity function and could not get away for that trip. We visited my cousin Heiner in Auckland, New Zealand, on our way to Melbourne.

If I have one regret about how the CINP has evolved, it is that the congresses have become too large, and are less and less conducive to interaction within small groups of academicians. This was possible in the early stages of the CINP when every second meeting was a closed meeting, not open to non-members. It has been an important part of my academic development and has allowed me to keep personal contact with leaders in the field whom I came to respect, and with many of whom I became friends. I look forward to the CINP to attract new members who will become leaders in the field in the decades to come.

Important psychopharmacological symposia were also held at several World Congresses of Psychiatry, Biological Psychiatry, and Pharmacology. I specifically remember the World Congresses in Montreal in 1961, and then in Madrid in 1966, when Linda and I also spent time in Spain visiting Seville, the Alhambra, and spent a week in Torremolinos at the Mediterranean near Málaga.

While in Madrid for the fourth World Congress, I organized and led a symposium on the effect of nonspecific or nondrug factors on drug and placebo response, the results of which were published in the book *Non-Specific Factors in Drug Therapy*, a publication still quoted today. Although biologically oriented, I always stressed and demonstrated the importance of a multifaceted, holistic approach to the pharmacological treatment of emotional illness. Linda and I stayed for two more weeks in Spain, sightseeing and relaxing at the beach. During this trip I also got to see my first bullfight.

I have fond memories of the 1961 World Congress of Biological Psychiatry held in Stockholm, which I visited with Crista and Larry, and combined it with a visit to Copenhagen; and of the congress in 1981, again, in Stockholm, where I led a symposium on benzodiazepine dependence. I also remember the one held in Philadelphia in 1985, when Linda and I arranged a big cocktail party, which was sponsored by the Department of Psychiatry, and held in the Rodin Museum. Larry and I visited Mexico City in 1972, and

Larry, my mother, and I visited Hawaii in 1977. Linda stayed home with Mike and Steve.

Our friends, the Freemans, joined us when we traveled to Florence, Venice, Nice, and another time to Athens, where we enjoyed a weeklong cruise. From Greece, Linda flew home with the Freemans, while I flew to Tokyo to extinguish some fires lit by employees of a large US pharmaceutical company. They had antagonized one of the leading Japanese psychiatrists and were planning to embarrass him even more in a public meeting two days later. I arranged for a private meeting with the psychiatrist, and we solved the problem between the two of us. At the next day's meeting I praised my Japanese colleague for the great work he had done, and apologized that I did not speak Japanese, a language my mother had studied at the Japanese embassy before the war in Berlin. During this visit I was also taken on a private tour of Kyoto. I can't help but wonder that this was yet again another example of serendipity and how we respond to it. Would I have gotten that rare and enjoyable experience in Kyoto if my intervention hadn't worked?

American College of Neuro-Psychopharmacology (ACNP)

Today probably the most influential and elite neuropsychopharmacology organization in the world is the American College of Neuropsychopharmacology (ACNP), founded in 1961. Its origin can be traced to a small meeting at the Barbizon Plaza Hotel in New York City in 1960, in which I also participated. The official organizational meeting of the College occurred at the Woodner Hotel in Washington, DC, in October 1961. The meetings were small and met for many years in Puerto Rico, first at the Sheraton and later at the larger Caribe Hilton. In these early days of psychopharmacology, all members and their spouses easily could fit in one picture, taken at the meeting's official dinner.

The annual meetings usually consist of one or two plenary sessions and several parallel panel sessions and study groups, some of which are held in the evening. For the first twenty years or so, the deliberations from each of these sessions were presented to the whole college at the end of the meeting. However, the most memorable interchange of ideas happened around the swimming pool, on the beach, or on the tennis courts or golf course. We poor scientists could not afford the winter rates in the Caribbean, and thus we met just the week before the winter rates went into effect, usually in the second week in December. Decades ago it was decided to have every fourth meeting on the West Coast, and it was usually held in Hawaii, but also in Acapulco and in Arizona. Linda came with me to these meetings only occasionally, as they were scheduled too close to Christmas and took time away from her Christmas preparations.

ACNP is world famous for its five volumes of the *Generation of Progress,* to which I contributed a chapter in each of the first four volumes. The fourth volume was published in 1995, and is more than two thousand pages long. These reviews, published each decade, provided the most up-to-date state of affairs in preclinical and clinical psychopharmacology at that time.

In later years, other countries started organizations representing the field too, but none as exclusive as the ACNP. I have been an active member for decades, participating or chairing study groups and panels. The best thing about this organization was that it brought together academic and NIMH staff and researchers, FDA officials, and industry researchers. Marketing people did not participate much in the meetings at that time.

Today the ACNP is still the most select organization in the field.

It is almost harder to become a member than to get into heaven (or hell, wherever your destination might be). While it started out very much with a clinical focus, it has evolved over the years into a multidisciplinary group, still only electing new members of the highest academic qualification.

Today some of the older members feel that the ACNP has become too much of a neuroscience meeting rather than a continuation of a meeting with more of a translational clinical focus. But no matter how you look at it, the ACNP has had a major impact on the study and development of psychopharmacology.

Early Clinical Drug Evaluation Unit (ECDEU)

The Psychopharmacology Service Center, under the leadership of Jonathan Cole, was established in the late 1950s by NIMH to manage research funding and to develop academic clinical psychopharmacological research units within America. Thus, the Early Clinical Drug Evaluation Unit (ECDEU) was started in 1959 and had its first meeting in 1960. I was there from its beginning.

About a dozen research centers received support from NIMH to further drug development methodology and to assure that only safe and effective drugs entered the American market. Some were at state hospitals and not at academic centers. Most of the units studied psychotic patients, while a few units studied depressed inpatients. Ours was the only unit that had independent NIMH support to study outpatient drug treatment in America. For ten years, one British unit also received NIMH support to evaluate drugs in family practice, using the practitioners as raters.

The early goal of the Psychopharmacology Service Center of NIMH was to encourage scientists and clinicians to enter the field, to develop interest in it, to find better drugs, and to develop a clinical trials methodology. ECDEU centers were run by well-trained researcher-clinicians who studied a small sample of patients intensively and shared their findings with other researchers in clinical psychopharmacology. Investigators, not industry, selected which drugs to study and when to publish the results. New potential therapeutic drug selection was determined by scientific curiosity, personal interest of the research group, public health interest, and advancement of clinical trial research methodology. Most of all clinical trial methodology was developed by NIMH-supported centers and groups in the '60s and '70s. Industry was only peripherally involved, if at all.

In the late 1970s, my NIMH-supported research turned to the problem of long-term benzodiazepine (BZ) use and BZ dependence, which can lead to withdrawal and other symptoms when benzodiazepines are abruptly discontinued. Low-dose dependence on benzodiazepines was recognized as a clinical problem, and over the next two decades our group provided many important research publications in this field. This interest of our group resulted in being invited to join the task force on benzodiazepine dependence established by the American Psychiatric Association.

The ECDEU met mostly at the Sonesta Hotel in Key Biscayne in the early years. But eventually the Sonesta became too small, and meetings were rotated among larger hotels in Florida, Arizona, California, and Nevada. We also met in New Orleans one year. During this meeting, Linda had to fly home early because one of the boys had become ill.

The ECDEU originally met twice yearly, and later, yearly. Most of these units were eventually closed, and in the early 1980s the name was changed to the New Clinical Drug Evaluation Unit (NCDEU). At that time, NIMH wanted the players in industry to fund their clinical drug development programs. While this was a reasonable suggestion, as federal funds were limited, drug development became, at least to some degree, more influenced by marketing forces than research departments, completely disregarding the continuation of methodological improvements. Because of this, my attendance at the meetings has become more sporadic. The growing influence of industry is a concern I just can't ignore. Today the majority of clinical trials that are sponsored by industry is conducted by private, not-university-affiliated, groups. Their motivation is not the promotion of scientific discovery, academic prestige, and the ability to publish the results of their work, but only financial rewards.

7

The Fiftieth Anniversaries of CINP and ECDEU

In 2008 and 2010 the first two scientific psychopharmacology organizations, established in 1958 and 1960, celebrated their fiftieth anniversaries. I had the pleasure and the honor to be present at both their births and their fiftieth anniversaries, not only as a spectator, but also as an invited speaker.

CINP 2008

The twenty-fifth CINP congress was held in Munich, Germany, in July 2008, and because the CINP holds congresses only every two years, it was also the fiftieth anniversary of the organization. Since I was one of the original clinicians who demonstrated the excellent anti-anxiety effects of the benzodiazepines, such as Librium and Valium, I was honored and thrilled to chair a scientific symposium entitled, "The Role of the Benzodiazepines in the 21st Century." Some of the world leaders in the field today joined me at this symposium, which was extremely well attended by hundreds of congress participants.

This event gave me an opportunity to think back on some of the important findings and discoveries in which I was fortunate to participate across half a century.

I had presented results of the first placebo-controlled study of Librium at the Pan-American Congress in Mexico City in 1960. Our group also studied diazepam against placebo long before the FDA approved it. We were able to conduct these controlled trials because we had NIMH grant support. Industry, at that time, would not support placebo-controlled trials. A few years later, when lorazepam was studied prior to FDA approval, again our group was involved.

For years, anxiety was (wrongly) considered a short-term, or intermittent, condition mostly observed in the "overworked house-wife." At that time psychoanalytic psychiatry in America felt that family physicians prescribed medication for everything from mild anxiety states that didn't need treatment, to more severe states, that should have been treated with psychotherapy. Yet, despite these views, Valium became the most prescribed medication in the world in the 1970s.

Over time it became apparent to psychiatrists that many patients were taking these anti-anxiety drugs for long periods of time. Such prolonged intake of a benzodiazepine (BZ) was considered at that time inappropriate, and great concern about over-prescribing was expressed in the media, before the US Congress, and particularly in Great Britain. Prolonged use of BZs became even more a concern when it was determined that many of these patients had great difficulties discontinuing the use of these drugs, particularly when stopping medication intake abruptly. This led to the informal definition of low-dose dependence on BZs. Interestingly enough, most patients did not increase the daily dosage of their BZ, yet still had difficulties stopping these drugs.

So, in the late '70s, our group became a worldwide recognized leader in studying this new phenomenon. Under NIMH grant support, we conducted the first placebo-controlled, double-blind study of long-term diazepam use, comparing the incidence and severity of abrupt discontinuation symptoms after six, twelve, and twenty-two weeks of diazepam treatment in anxious outpatients. This study was designed and submitted to NIMH in the mid-1970s, and reported in *JAMA* in 1983. We did a large series of studies in BZ dependence until the late 1990s, studying both the phenomenon as well as its treatment and management.

Double-Blind and Placebo Control

Perhaps I should explain what "double-blind" and "placebo control" mean. Placebo comes from the Latin word *to please* and refers to everything that may contribute to the study outcome, other than the medication. It includes the natural course of the illness, the belief that the doctor will help his patient, and many other factors such as treatment expectation, duration of illness, and other positive and negative events that may occur outside of the treatment situation. In the search for new treatments, we try to minimize such factors in order to assess the true medication effect, while in clinical treatment of our patients we like to encourage such placebo effects, because they may potentially boost the treatment outcome.

Double-blind means that for the weeks that the patient is in a study, neither the treating physician nor the patient will know whether the patient is on the active medication or the inert placebo. However, the drug code can be revealed at any time, particularly when the patient shows no improvement, experiences disturbing adverse events, or has just changed his mind and wants to stop being a patient in the research trial.

I was asked once why I never saw this dependence phenomenon in my private patients. I realized then that I was trained in medical school to prescribe medications under the following guidelines: "Increase slowly, attempt to get best results with as low a daily dose as possible, and always discontinue slowly," in other words "slow in, slow out." Thus, I always tapered my patients in the use of their BZ. When I studied long-term BZ users, I began to realize that these patients frequently were the sickest, often had secondary personality problems, and thus represented patients that today should be treated long-term.

While most experts today claim that antidepressants should be the first choice for the treatment of anxiety spectrum disorders, the fact is, even today, more prescriptions are written for BZs than antidepressants for anxiety disorders. Clearly the BZs still have an important role in treating anxiety disorders. They are also off patent and thus rather inexpensive.

Because BZs are so important for clinical practice, industry is searching for compounds that are similar to the BZs in efficacy, have an early onset of action, few adverse events, and less sedation and fewer discontinuation difficulties. Industry hoped to accomplish this fact by affecting certain gamma-aminobutyric acid (GABA) receptors selectively. Yet, so far, no such compound has been found.

A Changing Attitude

Since the first CINP congress, the academic community's view of anxiety has changed. While in the 1960s anxiety was considered by many not to be a real psychiatric illness, anxiety today is recognized as a chronic illness, often disabling, and in need of prolonged treatment. Had psychiatry looked at anxiety as a chronic illness earlier, the long-term treatment of anxious patients with drugs such as Valium might have been looked upon more positively. Comparing results from two of our long-term anxiety treatment trials, we found clear superiority for the BZ in early treatment up to eight weeks, but slightly better response with the antidepressant after six months of treatment. We determined that the BZ works swiftly, but reaches its maximal effect by four to eight weeks. Antidepressants on the other hand, even after four to eight weeks of treatment, have not yet reached their maximum improvement level. However, after six months of treatment, antidepressants may have a slight edge over the BZs. Whether this observation represented simply a chance finding or something more substantial, only a new, prospectively designed, controlled study could answer.

One day, before the twenty-fifth congress started, I attended a historical session entitled "View through Munich Psychiatry." The day started with a session and tour of the department of psychiatry at the Maximilian University and ended at the Max Planck, a national research institute. The two famous German psychiatrists constantly quoted were Kraeplin, the psychiatrist who for the first time distinguished between dementia praecox (schizophrenia) and manic-depressive illness, and Alzheimer, who first detected brain changes in demented patients.

Neither at the university nor at the Max Planck Institute did I ever hear the name Freud mentioned. This clearly is quite different from American psychiatry, where Freud's theory of personality still plays an important role in the teaching of our residents. One has to understand that German psychiatry is very much inpatient based, while psychiatry in America, even today, is very much outpatient based. Over the past forty years in Germany, psychotherapy was frequently taught and practiced in psychosomatic departments, often located within departments of internal medicine. However, in recent years this seems to have changed. Munich's department of psychiatry, for example, now has a psychotherapy section.

The twenty-fifth CINP congress was a highly personal experience for me. When I looked around at the president's dinner, a special event held in the Emperor's Hall at the residence of Bavaria's famous king, I saw only one person I remembered from the first congress in Rome. I had been one of the younger biological psychiatrists in 1958, so this wasn't a surprise. The friend whom I recognized as the only person being both in Rome in 1958, and now in Munich, was also the friend Linda and I skied with in St. Moritz in the early 1970s, while I was attending a depression conference held at the Suvretta House.

Controversy and Resolution

Over the years I have had much contact with German psychiatry, particularly with the Universities of Hamburg, the Free University of Berlin, and Munich University. I have given seminars and grand rounds at each. My German background made my advice desirable to German and Swiss pharmaceutical companies, as well as to German departments of psychiatry. My advice and appearance before the German FDA helped save the BZs, and particularly a short-half-life one, from being taken of the market.

I also was involved in the British lawsuits against Wyeth and Hoffmann la Roche, in which patients blamed the BZs not just for addiction but also for causing changes in personality and behavior. The British anti-BZ experts were lined up against US pro-BZ experts. I was one of the latter. The US group prevailed, and the high court in London ruled against the British experts.

Initially the marketers of BZs wanted to deny that their drugs could cause discontinuation symptoms. We advised strongly against such an approach and prevailed. We advised to admit that such difficulties do occur with prolonged treatment, followed by rather abrupt discontinuation, and advised to offer free "BZ discontinuation treatment," if necessary, in a hospital. But at the same time we advised the BZ manufacturers to fight all other claims, such as that a BZ caused divorces, personality problems, child abuse, and so on. We advised that such patients should be carefully examined by psychiatrists to assess whether or not the conditions prompting their complaints were preexisting. If so, then it could be stated that BZs were simply not effective in these patients, and probably should never have been used in these patients to begin with.

And, indeed, for all patients represented by the malpractice lawyers in England, it could be shown that their problems preceded the use of a BZ. And according to the British legal system, as I understand it, once the highest court had thrown these cases out, similar ones could not be filed again in lower courts. This closed an extremely large, expensive, and famous lawsuit in England. Wouldn't such a malpractice system be great also for America?

An interesting side note: while this lawsuit was being pressed, a BBC TV crew suddenly appeared at the Philadelphia Country Club. Both the president of Wyeth, the maker of Ativan, and I belonged to this club. The TV crew tried to get an interview with Wyeth's president, but when he refused, they followed him on the private golf course anyway to shoot pictures for British TV.

The British were (and still are) on a crusade against the BZs. Yet, when a few years ago I received a patient referral from one of the leading British BZ foes, what do you think his patient was taking as his psychiatric medication? You guessed it, a benzodiazepine. This, I believe, is a dangerous crusade. While I conducted a BZ discontinuation program at Penn, a medical resident referred to me a seventy-five-year-old woman who for more than ten years had been taking five milligrams of Valium once per day. She believed it was helping her, so I refused to take her BZ away. The referring resident was upset with me and on his own, replaced the five milligrams of Valium with seventy-five milligrams of imipramine, a first-generation antidepressant that also has anti-anxiety activity, but causes marked anticholinergic side effects.

Two to three months later I received a call from a surgical resident. He was working this woman up for an unknown abdominal tumor and preparing her for an exploratory operation. When I saw the patient I learned of her being placed on the antidepressant imipramine. My consultant report stated: "Please give an enema. Patient most likely has an impaction from the anticholinergic effects of imipramine." The bottom line was that I saved the elderly patient from a surgical intervention. Wasn't it much better for her to be on a low dose of diazepam (Valium) than on imipramine?

Another experience I had at about the same time focused on the use of short half-life hypnotic BZs. One of those short half-life hypnotics had caused tremendous problems in Holland for some patients, who became confused, psychotic, disoriented, and many other things. The makers of the drug asked me, a BZ expert who had also studied this drug, to fly to Brussels for an appearance before the Benelux authorities, an independent organization similar to our FDA. Imagine my surprise when I was introduced as "Dr. Rickels from XXX Company." Some of the members of the committee who knew me looked rather astounded.

I responded, "I am here to share with you my experience with this compound in question on the request of its maker, who also paid my travel expenses and a rather large honorarium. Most of you know me as an independent physician scientist from the University of Pennsylvania. My evaluation of the matter in question is that the manufacturer is fully to blame for what happened in Holland."

The manufacturer's representatives almost fainted and the whole room looked rather surprised. I then went into detail supporting my conclusion and came up with recommendations that if the drug were used at or below the dosage recommended in America, these serious adverse events would not have happened. The manufacturer's salesmen had recommended a dose up to eight times what was recommended in America. At a meeting held in Europe on another matter several months later, the chair of the committee to which I had appeared before pulled me aside and said, "Dr. Rickels, your honest presentation in Brussels a few months ago saved the drug from being taken off the market."

Discontinuation

As a proponent of the appropriate use of benzodiazepines, I'd like to take a couple of paragraphs here to summarize how I believe it is best to help a patient, when appropriate, to discontinue use of the medication. Discontinuation symptoms occur in about 40 to 60 percent of patients treated for four or more months, even after extended taper. They consist of a rebound of old anxiety and sometimes of the occurrence of new withdrawal symptoms, such as an increased acuity to sound and smell; symptoms peak during the end of taper and mostly will have disappeared in a few weeks. If they don't disappear, then it's very likely the patient still has anxiety or another psychiatric disorder.

The treatment is pretty straightforward. The first step is to establish a stable relationship between patient and physician. The second step is to aggressively treat, either with antidepressants or with cognitive therapy, any patient who still has anxious or depressive symptoms. The final step is to gradually taper the BZ dose over a three- to eight-week period after anxiety or depressive symptoms have been significantly reduced, while continuing the second treatment until the taper is concluded.

We concluded our symposium at the twenty-fifth congress with a reaffirmation that BZs represent a valuable group of medications. We concluded that they probably should be prescribed more frequently rather than less frequently. For treatment-resistant anxious patients, a combination of an antidepressant and a BZ might conceivably be the best approach, since both types of medication act via a different mechanism.

NCDEU 2010

The fiftieth anniversary of the NCDEU, formerly ECDEU, was held in June 2010 in Boca Raton, Florida. I had to postpone my trip to Greece, Italy, and Germany with my grandson, Andrew, for two weeks to be able to participate at the NCDEU meeting. I gave an invited lecture to several hundred participants entitled "Clinical Trial Methodology over Five Decades." I was one of the few current members who was also present at the first meeting of the ECDEU in 1960.

Thoughts on Methodology

A rather sobering conclusion drawn at the meeting was that almost all clinical trial methodology used today was developed in the 1950s and 1960s, long before industry became heavily involved in funding most drug trials. It was only updated later to reflect the newly developed American Psychiatric Association diagnostic criteria (DSM III, IIIR, IV).

I ended my presentation at the NCDEU congress by refuting the claims of industry, and also of some scientists, that an increase of the placebo response in psychiatric drug trials has occurred in the last twenty years, and that this, together with tougher FDA guidelines, has made it more difficult today to introduce new treatments for psychiatric disorders. I presented scientific data that clearly showed our group's placebo response, as well as that of other single-site academic research groups supported by the National Institutes of Health (NIH), had not changed during the past fifty years. I also stated that medications with robust effects could be detected today just as they were fifty years ago, and with many fewer patients per treatment group than industry uses today.

I believe strongly that the present problem with finding effective new psychiatric medications is caused basically by two factors. First, many new drugs studied today are simply not as effective as earlier drugs. For both clinician and researcher, it is important for their patients that a well-designed clinical trial allows a "good" drug not to fail, and a "weak" drug not to succeed. And, second, in order to save time, trial methodology employed by industry is negatively influenced today by their marketing, rather than positively by their research departments.

What contributes most likely to these failed trials? I believe there are five factors:

1. More and more inactive, or only mildly active, new compounds are being tested.

2. Clinical trials have moved from primarily academic centers to freestanding "for profit" practices. Primary motivation has shifted from scientific curiosity and academic advancement to financial gains.

3. Increasing sample sizes, up to two hundred patients per treatment arm, and increasing the number of study sites, from twenty to eighty, often in foreign countries not known for their clinical trial and psychiatric expertise. This clearly increases the variability or unreliability of the data collected.

4. Financial rewards for patient enrollment, including competitive enrollment, and not excluding questionable patients from the trial.

5. Study subjects are mostly advertised patients and professional patients, not true patients seen in the practices of family physicians or psychiatrists.

Many patients respond to advertising because of a temporary increase in their symptoms, often in response to an acute stress, and therefore should never be included into drug trials. Their symptom increase frequently improves simply with the passage of time.

Industry attempts to cope with their frequent inability, or at least difficulty, to differentiate drug from placebo by significantly enlarging the number of patients they are enrolling into a drug trial, and by introducing telephone, and even video, interviews; using independent raters (which frequently, in my opinion, at least, equals inexperienced raters); and using long, time-consuming, structured clinical interviews, all in the hope of increasing the sensitivity of their study, while, in my opinion, they may actually cause just the opposite.

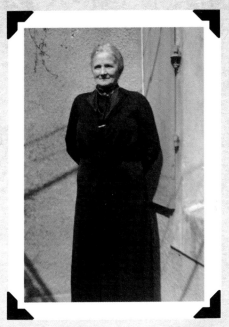

My father's mother, Gesche Maria (Harms) Rickels

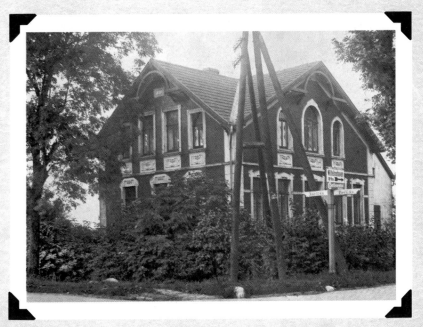

The family house in Sande, OST-Friesland, where my father grew up

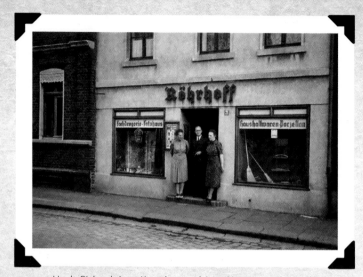

Uncle Richard, Aunt Kaetchen and Aunt Hanna stand outside
the house in Willich where my mother grew up

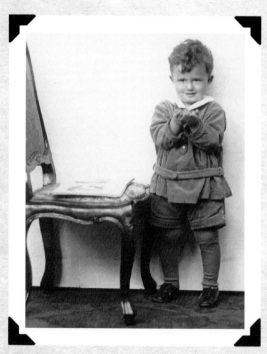

As a child in my Sunday suit

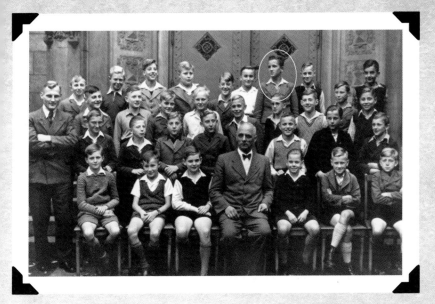

Gymnasium class picture, Grade 5 or 6, 1935 or 1936

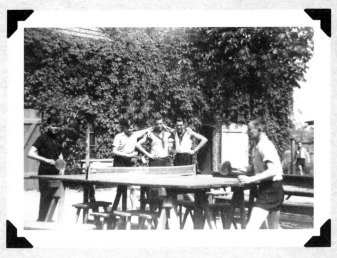

With classmates at the school camp in Tangersdorf

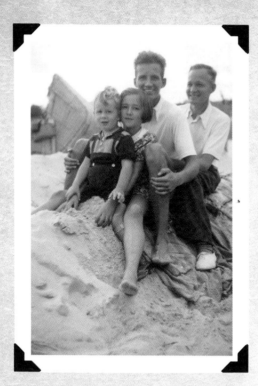

At the Baltic with my brother, Lothar, my sister, Gisela, and my father, 1940

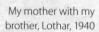

My mother with my brother, Lothar, 1940

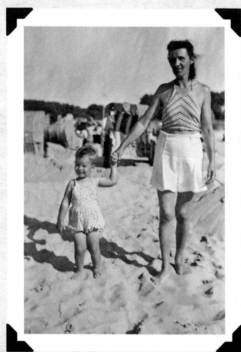

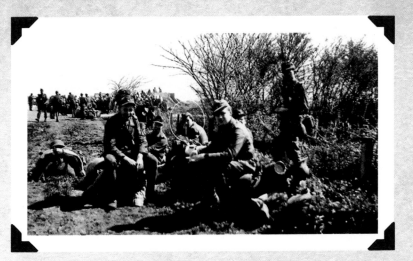

My first day of captivity in Africa, May 1943

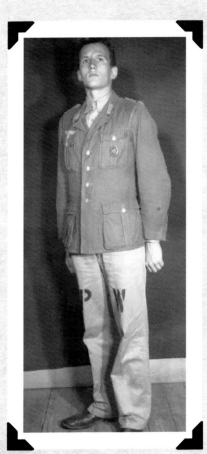

POW in America, 1945

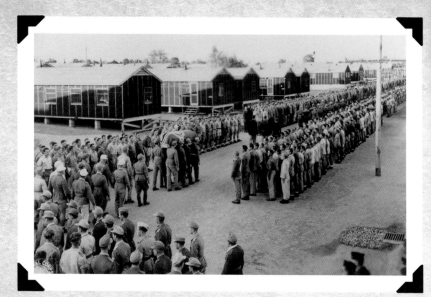

POW Camp Swift, Texas, 1944

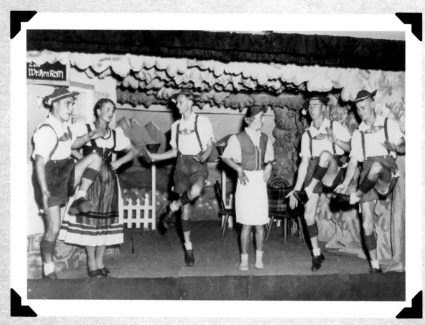

A show put on by prisoners, POW Camp Somerset, Maryland, 1944

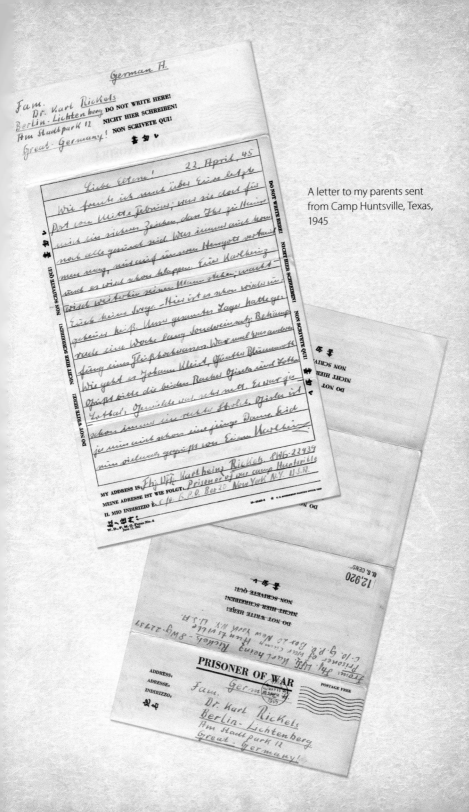

A letter to my parents sent from Camp Huntsville, Texas, 1945

Paid on the:
working-pay:
Discharge-pay:
Total:

B17438

CONTROL FORM D.2.
Kontrollblatt D.2.

B 1016

CERTIFICATE OF DISCHARGE
Entlassungschein

ALL ENTRIES WILL BE MADE IN BLOCK LATIN CAPITALS AND WILL BE MADE IN INK OR TYPESCRIPT.

I
PERSONAL PARTICULARS
Personalbeschreibung

Dieses Blatt **muss** in folgender weise ausgefüllt werden : 1. In lateinischer Druckschrift und in grossen Buchstaben. 2. Mit Tinte oder mit Schreibmaschine.

SURNAME OF HOLDER   RICKELS
Familienname des Inhabers

CHRISTIAN NAMES   KARL-HEINZ
Vornamen des Inhabers

CIVIL OCCUPATION   STUDENT (med)
Beruf oder Beschäftigung

HOME ADDRESS Strasse HOCHSTRASSE 21
Heimatanschrift Ort WILLICH
            Kreis KREFELD
            Regierungsbezirk/Land/.
            DUESSELDORF/RHEINLAND

DATE OF BIRTH 17.8.1924
Geburtsdatum (DAY/ MONTH/ YEAR)
            Tag/ Monat/ Jahr

PLACE OF BIRTH WILHELMSHAFEN
Geburtsort

FAMILY STATUS SINGLE   † Ledig
Familienstand MARRIED   Verheiratet
            WIDOW(ER)   Verwitwet
            DIVORCED   Geschieden

NUMBER OF CHILDREN WHO ARE MINORS
Zahl der minderjährigen Kinder NONE

I HEREBY CERTIFY THAT TO THE BEST OF MY KNOWLEDGE AND BELIEF THE PARTICULARS GIVEN ABOVE ARE TRUE.
I ALSO CERTIFY THAT I HAVE READ AND UNDERSTOOD THE "INSTRUCTIONS TO PERSONNEL ON DISCHARGE" (CONTROL FORM D.1).

Ich erkläre hiermit, nach bestem Wissen und Gewissen, dass die obigen Angaben wahr sind.
Ich bestätige ausserdem dass ich die ,, Anweisung für Soldaten und Angehörige Militär-ähnlicher Organisationen " u.s.w. (Kontrollblatt D.1) gelesen und verstanden habe.

SIGNATURE OF HOLDER
Unterschrift des Inhabers

KARL-HEINZ RICKELS

II
MEDICAL CERTIFICATE
Ärztlicher Befund

DISTINGUISHING MARKS SCAR ON THE FOREHEAD
Besondere Kennzeichen

DISABILITY, WITH DESCRIPTION NONE
Dienstunfähigkeit, mit Beschreibung

MEDICAL CATEGORY
Tauglichkeitsgrad

I CERTIFY THAT TO THE BEST OF MY KNOWLEDGE AND BELIEF THE ABOVE PARTICULARS RELATING TO THE HOLDER ARE TRUE AND THAT HE IS NOT VERMINOUS OR SUFFERING FROM ANY INFECTIOUS OR CONTAGIOUS DISEASE.

Ich erkläre hiermit, nach bestem Wissen und Gewissen, dass die obigen Angaben wahr sind, dass der Inhaber ungezieferfrei ist und dass er keinerlei ansteckende oder übertragbar Krankheit hat.

SIGNATURE OF MEDICAL OFFICER
Unterschrift des Sanitätsoffiziers

NAME AND RANK OF MEDICAL OFFICER IN BLOCK LATIN CAPITALS
Zuname/ Vorname/ Dienstgrad des Sanitätsoffiziers
(In lateinischer Druckschrift und in grossen Buchstaben)

JOHN E MILLER CAPT MC

P.T.O.
Bitte wenden

† DELETE THAT WHICH IS INAPPLICABLE
Nichtzutreffendes durchstreichen

LFF.   2159-12-45-500.000-79 673

Certificate of discharge by the British Occupation Forces

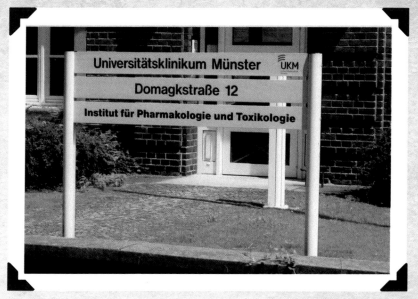

My medical school in Münster, Germany

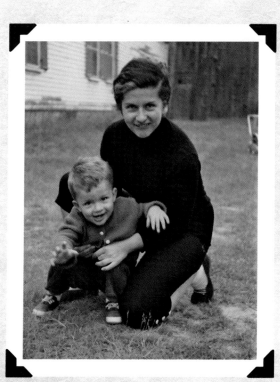

Crista and Larry, 1956

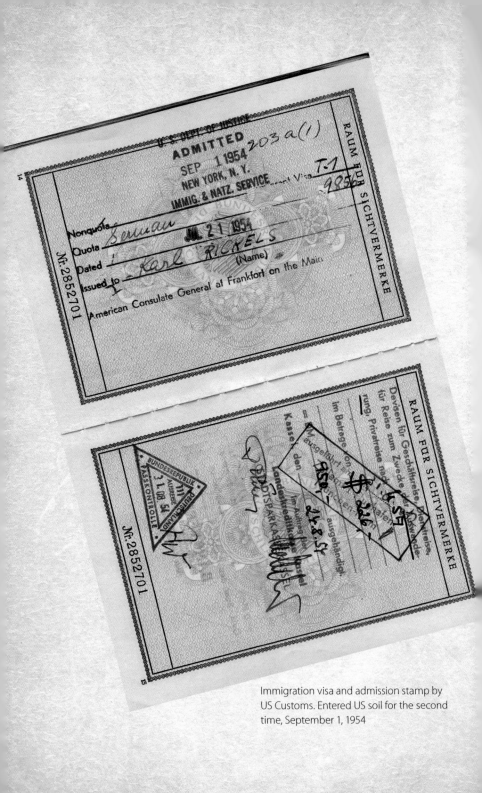

Immigration visa and admission stamp by US Customs. Entered US soil for the second time, September 1, 1954

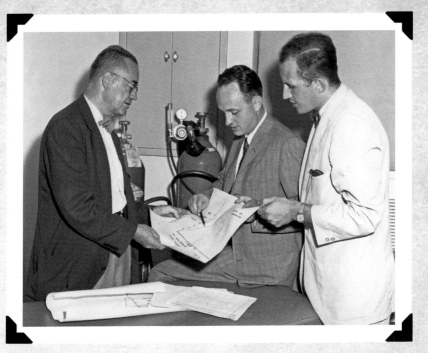

Dr. Appel, Chair of Psychiatry, Dr. Ewing and myself, 1956

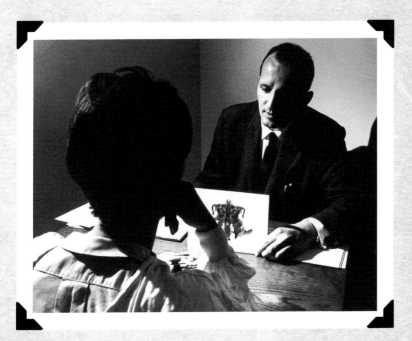

Administering an inkblot test to a patient, 1957

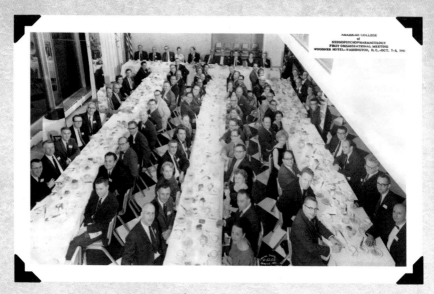

Inauguration of ACNP in Washington, DC, 1961

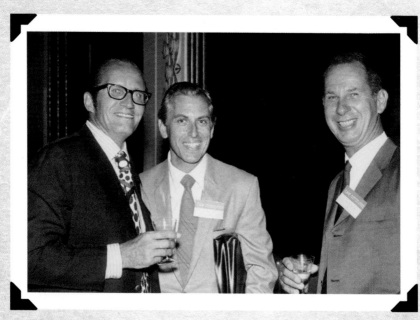

With two of my oldest colleagues and friends, Dr. Levine and Dr. Hollister

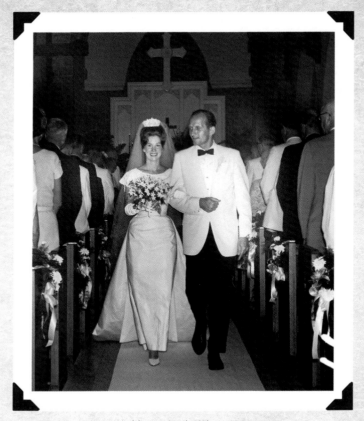

Wedding to Linda Wilson, 1964

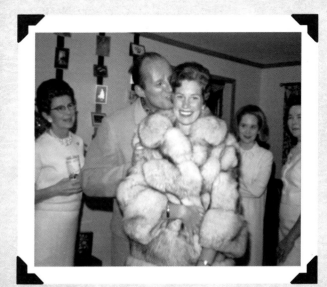

New Year's Eve party,
late 1960's

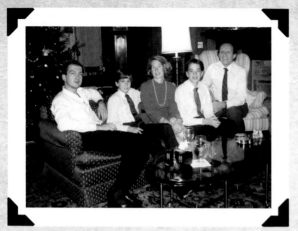

Christmas at Sweetbriar
with Larry, Mike, Linda
and Steve

In my office at Penn

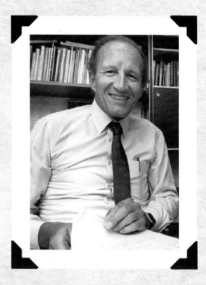

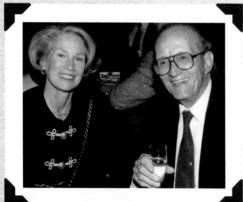

Linda and Karl

CHRISTMAS 2007

"Angels from the realms of glory wing your flight o'er all the earth …"

With Christmas Greetings

We have had a delightful Thanksgiving with Larry and Ellie, and Heidi and Steve. **Larry** is off to Berlin for Christmas with Ellie in tow. But never fear, he should be back to teach at Santa Barbara by February.

Steve and **Heidi** have been busy this past year. We threw a party for them in March here in Gladwyne so that our eastern friends would have a chance to get to know Heidi. We were lucky and Ricki and Johnny were here for the occasion too. What fun! Just to keep us off balance, Steve and Heidi moved to a new home in Indian Hills, CO. Guess what comes with a new home? Heidi is expecting a baby in early May! I wonder what Nico thinks about the new situation??

Alyssa and **Mike** still love the city and their cottage in Eaglesmere. Personal use has become a new prime priority. Andrew (now 9) is a nice athlete. Soccer and baseball are favorite pastimes just now. Peter (6) is my dreamer and follows Andrew most of the time. Claudia and Caroline (3) continue to be mobile, high energy, verbal, and the most adorable rascals of little girls one could ever see. Kudos to Alyssa! Between her work at church and counseling at Pennsylvania Hospital, I don't know how she does everything! Mike just loves his work and academia.

Although **Karl** still works fulltime at Penn, he enjoyed skiing with Mike and "the Boys" in Wyoming in late March. Karl also did escape with his two grandsons and me to Williamsburg for a long weekend over our anniversary. We saved a trip for September, and went to China. We had a wonderful 2weeks in a world that was totally new to us. This year I've been busy furnishing the "new" rooms in our home, as well as, the terrace and flower gardens. It's been delightful to have this area back in our lives. Thanksgiving is over and now it's time to decorate in order to be ready for Christmas.

It's been lonely without Mother. I still miss her tales and her wonderful sense of humor Her friend Karl Parrish died a month ago. Now they can be together again.

"..........Come and worship, come and worship; Worship Christ the newborn King."
Words by James Montgomery· Music by Henry Smart

Love and best wishes,

Linda and Karl

SEASON'S GREETINGS

Linda's last Christmas letter

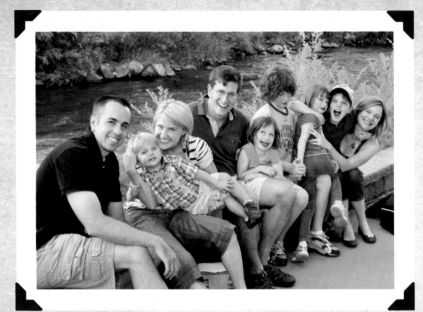

Steve and Mike with their wives and families

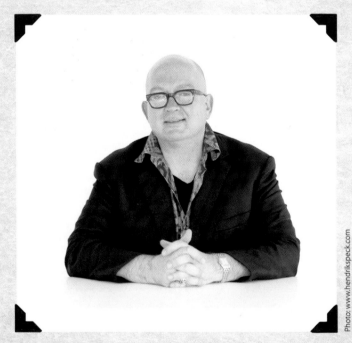

Larry at The European Graduate School

Paper texture: iStockphoto.com

Photo: www.hendrikspeck.com

I believe that the response of patients to a prolonged interview and to extended times spent in the research clinic can be divided into two categories. Patients either like the extra time spent at the clinic, often experiencing a high placebo response, or they hate it, frequently lowering both the placebo and drug response. Since both types of patients are usually enrolled into a drug trial, their treatment responses contribute to a narrowing of active drug-placebo differences, resulting in what we call an enlarged error rate, and an increased insensitivity to detect treatment differences. The approaches described above have provided financial gains, however, not to the industry who sponsors and supports a clinical trial, but to the clinical research organizations (CROs), which make more money the more patients they monitor; to the organizations that provide rater training, as well as patient ratings by telephone or video, irrespective of whether these activities are helpful; and, finally, to the many study sites involved in such a trial.

What can we do to improve today's clinical trial designs favored by industry? I recommend to return to designs used for several decades in mostly NIH-supported trials. That would mean the following:

1. Reintroduce a single site, or at the most two- to six-site multicenter trials, with each site contributing at least fifty patients.
2. Reduce treatment group sample sizes to, at the most, fifty patients.
3. Decrease reliance on advertised patients and on chronic trial or for-money patients, and shift to obtaining psychiatric study patients from family and psychiatric practices.

4. Increase involvement of academia in the design and conduct of drug efficacy trials. Create a number of NIH-funded Centers of Excellence in academia, with sufficient federal funding, so that these centers can function financially independent from industry support. Such academic centers would allow the conduct of swift and efficient, small sample size, efficacy trials of new and innovative agents.

This approach would, in my opinion, provide a natural path to personalized medicine, and would speed up the introduction of new, innovative, and better psychiatric medications to help our patients.

The anniversaries of the CINP and NCDEU are milestones in the still young field called psychopharmacology. I'm honored to have been a part of these organizations from the beginning. But the task today is the same as it was fifty years ago: we need new and better ways to treat our patients, not just "me too" medications. We need new and daring approaches. Our patients deserve it!

8

My Personal Contributions to the Field

It is most exciting to me that I started in psychiatry at the time when old, ineffective psychiatric treatments were replaced by new ones, namely medications, and that I was allowed to assist at the birth of this new science, called psychopharmacology, a science that focuses on the study of the effects of various medications on the psyche, and particularly on emotional or psychiatric symptoms. All my research over the past decades was influenced by an overriding interest to find better treatments for my patients with emotional and psychiatric symptoms.

My main research interest in all these years focused on the treatment of nonpsychotic outpatients suffering from anxiety and/or depression. This group represents by far the largest group of psychiatric patients often first treated by their family physician. But anxiety disorders occupied my research interest preferentially for a long time. I will touch shortly on several areas of research that occupied me for decades. Before I do so, however, I need to mention that since clinical trial methodology was in its infancy in 1955, all my research also included a focus on the improvement of trial methodology.

Penn Clinical Psychopharmacology Research Unit

I established the Penn Clinical Psychopharmacology Research Unit in 1959 with a primary focus on anxiety disorders, depression, insomnia, and research methodology. For many years it has been considered one of the leading outpatient research units in the world. The unit was prominent in the early developments of meprobamate and later of the benzodiazepines, Librium, Valium, Ativan and Xanax. In later years, buspirone (Buspar), the first non-benzodiazepine anxiolytic, entered the market, based largely on our studies. And, in the late 1970s and early 1980s, the findings by our group that antidepressants are also effective in the treatment of anxiety quickly encouraged industry to study all second-generation antidepressants in anxiety disorders.

We also conducted many studies of older and newer antidepressants, studies that were often considered pivotal by the FDA for the drug approval process. Most of this research was supported by research grants from the NIMH. My first NIMH grant started in 1959 (MH-02934), and my last NIMH grant ended December 2009 (MH-65063). One of my research grants (MH-08957) ran for thirty-two years, the longest duration of any NIMH research grant that I am aware of.

Non-Specific Factors in Treatment Response

One of my many early research interests was the improvement of methodology, an unexplored field in clinical research in the 1950s and 1960s. I became intensely interested in what factors other than the drug affected the patient's treatment outcome. The role that nonspecific factors play in the drug and placebo response in outpatients became my main research interest for a long time and led to my chairing a symposium on this topic at the 1966 World Congress of Psychiatry in Madrid. Again, although biologically oriented, I always stressed in my teachings and publications the importance of a multifaceted, holistic approach to the pharmacological treatment of emotional symptoms.

Satellite Outpatient Clinical Trial Network

Created in the early 1960s, this was the first satellite community research center in the world. I moved clinical research from tertiary and charity hospital clinics into private family and private psychiatric practice on the premise that drug and placebo responses should be studied in populations where these illnesses (depression and anxiety disorders) are primarily present and recognized. This development served as a model for today's multicenter trials in psychiatry, and was a forerunner by decades of today's interest in effectiveness research in the community. Even today I still conduct my major research in several family practices in the Philadelphia area.

Low Dose Benzodiazepine Dependence

In the late 1970s my group's research focus turned to benzodiazepine dependence and its management. Our group quickly became one of the most recognized and productive groups in the world on this topic. This led to travel to many countries in Europe, as well as South Africa, Hong Kong, Australia, Japan, and many other places.

NIMH-Sponsored Collaborative Research
in Anxious Outpatients

I was extremely honored when Sey Fisher, PhD, an associate of Jonathan Cole, MD, head of the Psychopharmacology Service Center at NIMH, invited Dr. E. H. Uhlenhuth from Johns Hopkins (Uhli, to his friends) and me to join him in a program to study the role of expectations on drug response in anxious outpatients. This was in 1960, a time when collaborative research was still in its infancy. Our program was the first outpatient collaborative study ever supported by NIMH. It involved three academic centers, the Psychopharmacology Service Center of NIMH, Johns Hopkins University, and the University of Pennsylvania.

Our collaborative research was conducted over a period of twelve years ("Outpatient Study of Drug/Set Interaction," MH04731). Many methodologically important publications resulted from our work. The first two collaborative studies focused on the interaction between treatment setting and drug and placebo treatment response in anxious outpatients. At some point we were joined by Ronald Lipman, PhD, from NIMH, and Lino Covi, MD, from Johns Hopkins.

In one study we showed that doctors expressing a positive, enthusiastic therapeutic attitude toward medication produced in their patients a higher drug and a lower placebo response than doctors trained to express an uncertain, experimental attitude. In another methodologically-oriented study, we explored the effect of a positive versus neutral interpretation of "dry mouth" produced by atropine on the treatment response to Librium or placebo. To our surprise, we learned that patients did not accept our "positive" association of the side effect dry mouth with positive treatment response. In the patients' own words, dry mouth was considered a bad side effect without any positive connotation. This was quite in contrast to findings of another study in which patients attributed sedation with a positive connotation, particularly if it helped them to sleep. This collaborative research program also led to the development of one of the most widely-used-patient-completed rating scales in the world, the Hopkins Symptom Checklist.

NIMH-PRB Pharmacotherapy of Anxiety and Depression

In 1973, Douglas McNair, a PhD from Boston University and developer of the Profile of Mood States (POMS), joined our group. We had shifted our research focus to the treatment of depression with anxiolytics and of anxiety with antidepressants. NIMH supported the program from 1974 to 1981 (MH-26025). We observed that while anxiolytics, chlordiazepoxide in this case, were ineffective in treating depression, the antidepressant imipramine (Tofranil) indeed demonstrated anxiolytic efficacy, more so in fact than the benzodiazepine. Results from this study certainly brought into question the widely held belief that antidepressants were ineffective in the treatment of anxiety.

This led to a second NIMH-supported study ("Antidepressants in the Treatment of Anxiety," MH-40000), conducted by our group with patients suffering from generalized anxiety disorder (GAD). After eight weeks of treatment, imipramine was found to be slightly more effective than diazepam, while diazepam was clearly the treatment of choice during the first two weeks of treatment. Our research on the effectiveness of imipramine in GAD led eventually to a series of industry-supported, large multicenter clinical trials to study marketed antidepressants in the treatment of anxiety. This research is frequently cited as an example of how federally funded research can stimulate new treatment discoveries by industry.

The Past Ten Years

In the last decade, academia has focused increasingly on improving the treatment of patients with a treatment-resistant psychiatric illness. Academia has been striving more and more to learn how to help the patient to reach remission, a symptom-free state. In order to reach a symptom-free state, patients frequently have to be treated for prolonged periods of time, try out several different medications, combine several medications, or be treated with a combination of drug and non-drug psychotherapies. This has led us to the newest goal in medicine, not only in psychiatry, but in all fields: personalized medicine. New research into such areas as pharmacogenetics offers us hope that we may eventually be able to personalize the treatment of our patients.

Research Program in Women's Health

In the late 1960s and 1970s, as part of the development of the Hopkins Symptom Checklist (HSCL), I expanded its use into family practice. I studied its sensitivity and specificity in assessing mild levels of emotional symptomatology, which, by itself, may not qualify for a full psychiatric major diagnosis, but still produces enough temporary symptom distress that could affect the patient's quality of life.

During that time, Celso Garcia, MD, a leading infertility expert and surgeon, who was one of the co-developers of the birth control pill, came from Boston to Philadelphia. Soon Linda became his infertility patient, after we tried for an extended period of time to have a baby. Dr. Garcia performed a tuboplasty operation on Linda's Fallopian tubes to open them up. Dr. Garcia and I soon found out that we had similar research interests. My interest in the use of the HSCL in non-psychiatric populations, and my expertise in assessing changes in anxious and depressed patients, irrespective of the methods with which they had been treated, was just what Celso needed to widen the research activities in the Obstetric-Gynecology department.

A new collaboration, lasting for decades, was born. Certainly, had Linda and I not had some infertility problems, Dr. Garcia and I might have never gotten together in our research. Again, as so often was the case in my life, serendipity, or fate, clearly guided and helped me. We established a Women's Health Program, which I took over as its leader about a decade later with the establishment of the Mudd Professorship Program, its income supporting part of the program. Most support, however, came from NIH, and, particularly in the beginning, from several foundations.

The program first focused on the emotional health in Ob-Gyn patients, the psychological impact of abortion on the woman, on lactation suppression, post-coital contraception, the morning-after pill, and oral contraception, showing that estrogen, but not progesterone, had moderate antidepressant properties. We then extended into the infertility area, studying anovulatory women and the emotional distress related to infertility, and its treatment.

Dr. Emily Mudd, who had established the first marriage council agency in Pennsylvania, had just retired and joined our group and brought with her a young PhD in social sciences from Bryn Mawr College, Dr. Ellen Freeman. We extended our program, largely focusing on the emotional, psychological, and social well-being of never-pregnant teenagers, as well as those with unwanted teen pregnancy. We also conducted a school program to prevent teenage pregnancy. Dr. Freeman and I wrote up our main results in a book entitled, *Early Childbearing: Perspectives of Black Adolescents on Pregnancy, Abortion, and Contraception.* We found that present emotional status and future schooling and work opportunities were greatly enhanced in the two groups of teens who either never got pregnant or who chose to abort their first pregnancy, compared to those teens who decided to carry their pregnancy to term and to raise their babies.

This program was continuously supported by NIH, but also by the Pew and Grant Foundations. Dr. Freeman and I shifted our research interest to the study and treatment of premenstrual symptoms (PMS). This research has been continuously supported by NIH for twenty-five years (HD186330), and has been the only PMS-treatment grant awarded by NIH. Dr. Freeman is today considered one of the leading researchers in the world in PMS. I am extremely proud and happy to have been Dr. Freeman's mentor in the past and her friend ever since.

Books, Peer-Reviewed Research Publications, Reviews, and Book Chapters

Reviewing my publication records, I find that I have published or edited nine books, starting with *Non-Specific Factors in Drug Therapy,* which was published in 1968, and ending with *Good Chemistry,* published in 2004. In addition, I have published more than 580 scientific papers, reviews, and book chapters.

9

Reflections on Psychopharmacology Today

Being a psychiatrist and psychiatric researcher for more than fifty years, my main overarching goal has always been to find improved treatments for my patients. The birth of psychopharmacology was an exciting period for psychiatry and for me personally. Over a ten-year period in the 1950s and early 1960s, almost all classes of medications used for today's treatment of most psychiatric illnesses were developed. There existed no such treatments before.

Early Psychopharmacology

From 1954 to 1964, I had the great fortune to work in psychiatry when, for the first time, effective treatments for mental illnesses became available. And while during the first half year of my training I still experienced the old psychiatry, with psychotic patients being treated with strait jackets, cold water, electroshock, insulin coma, and transorbital lobotomies, after six months I saw with my own eyes the tremendous benefits of the new antipsychotic medications, chlorpromazine (Thorazine) and reserpine (Serpasil).

These new psychiatric medications were all discovered by a combination of serendipity and astute clinical observation, not by controlled trials, and not based on molecular or neurotransmitter theories. Presumed mechanisms of action for most of these drugs were not discovered until many years after they were introduced into psychiatry.

The first neuroleptic, chlorpromazine (Thorazine), used to treat schizophrenia, was studied as an antihistamine for sedation. The first tricyclic antidepressant, imipramine (Tofranil), was tested in schizophrenia where it was ineffective, but, surprisingly, it showed mood elevating properties. The first monamine oxidase inhibitor (MAOI), iproniazid (Marsalid), originally a treatment for tuberculosis, was found to possess mood-elevating properties. The first drug discovered for the treatment of manic-depressive illness (bipolar disorder) was lithium. It was first used in the 1940s in Australia, yet it took more than twenty years to establish its mood-stabilizing effect worldwide. Lithium is still the mainstay in the treatment of this illness. In the early 1960s, astute clinicians observed the mood-stabilizing effects of several anticonvulsants, offering alternatives to lithium. Methylphenidate (Ritalin) and other stimulants, studied for treating fatigue, were found to be excellent treatments for treating attention deficit hyperactivity disorder (ADHD). For over 50 years Ritalin is still the standard for treating ADHD in children as well as in adults.

The very short half-life drug mephenesin, originally tested in the laboratory to provide a longer half-life for penicillin, was found in mice to possess muscle relaxant properties. Frank Berger made the connection between muscle relaxation and anxiety and developed mephenesin's longer half-life derivative, meprobamate (Miltown), as the first minor tranquilizer, replacing the barbiturates.

The benzodiazepines, chlordiazepoxide (Librium) and diazepam (Valium), were discovered a few years later when a series of compounds was screened in the laboratory for any type of possible pharmacological effect.

New drug development since that time has stalled. Most new drugs are basically "me too" drugs. Though they typically have a different side-effect profile, there is little or no improved efficacy. These second-generation drugs are possibly safer, but no more efficacious than first generation medications. Our tremendous scientific laboratory advances, such as those made in the fields of molecular sciences and nanotechnology, have, regretfully, at least in psychiatry, not yet led to new treatments working via completely new mechanisms.

In the double-blind studies carried out in the 1960s and 1970s, at a time when industry just began to get interested in controlled studies, and when most placebo-controlled studies were still conducted under NIMH support, treatment differences between active drug and placebo were discovered with sample sizes of less than fifty per treatment group. Frequently, only thirty patients per treatment group were needed to demonstrate superiority of drug over placebo.

In contrast, today drug-placebo differences are frequently smaller when studying these newer agents, demanding much larger sample sizes to demonstrate statistical, even if not clinically meaningful, drug efficacy. I am not sure which is the cart and which is the horse. Is it that newer drugs are less effective and therefore a study needs a large patient sample size to demonstrate efficacy, or does the fact that industry's use of large numbers of patients from many study sites to conduct a drug trial faster creates such large variability in the study sample that it is hard to demonstrate treatment differences? In either case, only side-effect profiles and excessive marketing, not efficacy, differentiate the newer from the older compounds.

The New and the Old

In my clinical experience, the newer antidepressants, such as fluoxetine (Prozac), paroxetine (Paxil), sertraline (Zoloft), venlafaxine (Effexor) and others have shown to be particularly helpful in the treatment of minor depressions, and in major depressions when used for prolonged periods of time. The older antidepressants, such as imipramine (Tofranil) and amitriptyline (Elavil), work at least equally well in depressed patients, but severe dry mouth and other anticholinergic and sedative side effects frequently keep patients from taking them regularly. Daily dosage adjustment is also slightly more difficult with the older than with the second-generation antidepressants. Perhaps most importantly, a weekly dose could allow a suicidal patient to kill himself with the older antidepressants through overdose. In contrast, the second-generation antidepressants are safer in this regard, but cause other, often equally disturbing, side effects, such as gastrointestinal symptoms, dizziness, and sexual dysfunction.

Similarly, the newer neuroleptics (antipsychotics) such as risperidone (Risperdal), olanzapine (Zyprexa), quetiapine (Seroquel) and others differ from the older ones such as the phenothiazines (Thorazine and others) and haloperidol (Haldol) only in their side-effect profile, exchanging anticholinergic and antihistamine adverse events and tardive dyskinesia (involuntary mouth and tongue movement), with excessive weight gain and pre- or full-type 2 diabetes.

Only many years later did we learn that antipsychotics work primarily via the dopamine system, and even much later that the serotonergic system is also involved. Most antidepressants are now considered to work primarily via the serotonergic and noradrenergic systems, and the benzodiazepines via the GABA-A system. Over the years many different subunits of the GABA-A receptor have been discovered, yet none of these discoveries has yet produced a better anxiolytic than the benzodiazepines. Similarly many types of serotonin receptors have been identified, although their study has not yet led to better antidepressants or anxiolytics.

Thus, by the mid-1960s we had almost all medications available to treat most psychiatric illnesses responsive to medication.

Much later, in the early 1980s, buspirone (Buspar), a serotonin IA partial agonist, was introduced by our group as the first and only non-BZ anxiolytic ever marketed. However, it was less effective than the BZs, worked much more slowly, and was void of any sedative effect, an effect anxious patients often desire in their medication, as frequently they have marked sleep problems. Yet, it caused no withdrawal symptoms, even after abrupt discontinuation, and can be taken with alcohol, while the BZs cannot. This fact often influenced the choice of anxiolytic I would prescribe in my private practice. Buspirone has also been shown to have antidepressant properties, yet its clinical use has always been rather limited. Soon good clinicians observed that antidepressants are also excellent anti-anxiety agents.

From a historical perspective, even more astounding is the fact that the discoveries in the '50s and early '60s were made with a much smaller financial investment and fewer researchers than today. Today we focus a great deal on drug-drug interactions, mostly related to how cytochrome P450 liver enzymes affect drug metabolism, or how these enzymes affect the metabolism of other medications. Yet, when one of the first drug-drug interactions was discovered between Tagamet, an antiacid, and Valium, our solution was simple: reduce the Valium dose slightly when also prescribing Tagamet for peptic ulcer.

Today, many of us are enthralled with the concept of comorbidity and diagnostic purity. Every little symptom is a comorbid, or independent, psychiatric illness. The anxiety in major depression or in major psychosis is comorbid, generalized anxiety disorder. In my view, real comorbidities would be diseases such as diabetes and schizophrenia, or alcohol misuse and another psychiatric disorder, but not generalized anxiety disorder and social phobia or panic disorder, or even depression.

The Growing Influence of Marketing

Today the marketing departments in the pharmaceutical industry are more powerful than ever. Consumer marketing is en vogue, yet is allowed only in very few countries besides the US. Many physicians feel that the FDA should disallow such advertising. It also appears at times as if medical leaders, academicians and non-academicians alike, willing as well as unwilling, represent more the interests of industry than of their patients.

For example, when a large pharmaceutical company developed a new group of BZs—the triazolo BZs and particularly the short half-life derivative, alprazolam (Xanax)—the manufacturer had to look for a new diagnostic indication. Non-psychotic anxiety or generalized anxiety disorder was no longer a profitable diagnosis. Thus, the manufacturer and a group of academicians created a new diagnosis, *panic disorder*. Some of the early diagnostic criteria included that if a patient had only one panic attack in a month he would be diagnosed with generalized anxiety disorder, but if he had more than one panic attack in a month, he would be diagnosed with panic disorder. Does this make clinical sense?

Two large-scale, international, multicenter studies were conducted and a new psychiatric diagnosis was born. The implication was that the older BZs would not be helpful in this disorder. This was believed by most clinicians the world over, yet it was simply not true. Older BZs, when prescribed in somewhat higher daily dosages, were equally effective in treating panic disorder as Xanax. I was one of a very few academicians who said so from the beginning, and was, therefore, invited at an upcoming ECDEU meeting to address the role of older BZs for the treatment of panic disorder. Since all older BZs, such as diazepam (Valium) and lorazepam (Ativan), were introduced into the market for neurotic anxiety disorders, a classification that included patients with panic symptoms, no panic-specific studies ever needed to be done for registration. All anxiety disorders were subsumed under one diagnosis.

Soon thereafter, industry and a select group of academic psychiatrists and psychologists created the next new psychiatric diagnosis. They named this new illness *generalized social phobia,* symptoms until then subsumed under nonpsychotic anxiety disorders.

It is most interesting that these two new psychiatric diagnoses were created to enlarge the profits of two very strange bedfellows: the pharmaceutical industry, which markets second-generation antidepressants as well as selected BZs for these disorders, and cognitive behavioral psychotherapists, who benefit from a new income stream for cognitive therapy. I suggest that it is now time, in this new millennium, to return to the diagnostic guidance offered more than one hundred years ago by Freud, and combine again the three anxiety diagnoses into one, separating out only patients with severe phobic symptoms.

Finally, post-traumatic stress disorder (PTSD), an appropriate psychiatric diagnosis, is considered by many to be an overused diagnosis, providing more financial rewards to the therapists, than symptom relief to their patients.

Most academic advisors to industry today are advisors to marketing departments and not, as in my time, to research departments. Also, today academia is highly represented on the speakers' bureaus of industry, pushing the new and financially rewarding patented compounds, and using industry-provided slides for very rewarding speaker fees. I have never participated in these speakers' bureaus. I have always felt that my research should speak for itself. In my opinion, today, academia, which is so dependent on pharmaceutical funding and consulting fees, is overvaluing the newer medications and undervaluing the older ones, which have by now become generic and therefore are less expensive than the patent-protected, mostly "me too," prescription drugs.

A few years ago when fellows in internal medicine at the Hospital of the University of Pennsylvania became aware that their rather poor patients could not afford to buy the expensive newer antidepressants prescribed to them by the young doctors, I advised them to prescribe imipramine (the first tricyclic antidepressant ever developed). For that year, depressed patients were treated in the medical clinic with imipramine and experienced significant improvement in their depressive symptoms, all thanks to a medication they could actually afford.

Research Valued by FDA and Industry

Almost all of the studies I've been involved in were later considered "pivotal" by the FDA in its approval process. In fact the latest antidepressant, vilazodone, was just approved by the FDA in January 2011 for the treatment of adult depression, based on a pivotal study to which my group significantly contributed. One other of my main contributions to the industry's development of new drugs was that I was able to shoot down many ineffective compounds early in their development, saving hundreds of millions of dollars. When "The Rickels Group," as our research group was being referred to worldwide, found early on that a drug appeared to be ineffective, this almost always held up in future clinical trials, and the same was true when we found a drug effective. For decades the findings of our research clinic, including our family practice satellite clinics, became the barometer for the FDA and industry to judge the sensitivity of drug development of all anxiolytics and antidepressants.

Let me digress for a moment. When I was approached by the FDA in the early 1970s to take over as chair of a review panel of over-the-counter sedatives, calmatives, and stimulants, I hoped to get out of this time-consuming job by stating that I had a number of conflicts of interests. I mentioned that I had several large NIMH grants to manage, that I was a consultant to many research divisions of national and international pharmaceutical companies, and had conducted several large-scale medication trials over the past year. When the FDA lawyer asked me to clarify my statements, and particularly asked me to reveal how many studies turned out positive and how many negative, it just so happened that all but one clinical trial had been negative over the previous year. At this point, the lawyer responded, "You have the job. With such a track record we will easily defend you at any time that US Congress should raise any questions about conflicts of interest." And so I was committed to three years of part-time public service.

Psychopharmacology and Psychotherapy

It is my experience, gained over many decades, that the addition of some kind of psychotherapy—combining psychodynamic, behavioral, cognitive, and interpersonal approaches—to medication therapy represents the best approach to treat most psychiatric illnesses, especially if provided by the same therapist. This is the approach I have employed over many decades of private practice. While drugs are clearly the best choice for the acute treatment of seriously ill patients, the addition of psychotherapy, used in the broadest sense, frequently leads to better long-term outcome and fewer relapses.

In my experience, some of the benefits psychotherapy adds to medication therapy are the following:

1. It helps the patient deal more effectively and realistically with the stress that triggers his/her anxiety and depression;
2. It teaches the patient to interpret cues accurately so he or she can learn from negative, as well as positive, cues;
3. It helps the patient adjust to life with all its many imperfections, and learn to see the kernel of good, even in the most painful situation; and
4. It teaches the patient to never lose hope.

In other words, the goal of psychotherapy is teaching the patient to help him/herself. In this process our drugs are merely tools and not a panacea. I realized early in my career that a treatment approach has to be tailored to the patient's need, not the need of the treating psychiatrist.

No one is more aware than I that even the physician who is not knowingly providing psychotherapy is providing some psychotherapeutic support, even if unwittingly. Therefore, any results that we obtain with medication include not only the pharmacological effect of the medication, but also the placebo effect any physician-patient contact entails. When I treat a patient in a clinical setting, I like to have as much placebo response as possible, as this effect is additive to the medication effect. On the other hand, in clinical *research* I try to lower the placebo effect as much as possible in order to more clearly delineate the medication's effect from the placebo effect.

I learned very early in my career that the main difference between family physicians who are successful with their use of psychiatric medications and those who are not is three to five minutes, the time needed to introduce the medication appropriately to the patient. Presented as a tool to help the patient, instead of a cure-all or panacea, the treatment is more likely to be successful.

Even today, in my old age, I still enjoy being with my patients and helping them with their psychiatric problems. And my patients do like me and respond to my interventions. It is nearly impossible, however, to develop the kind of relationship and rapport that I have with my patients within the twenty minutes allowed by most insurances.

Not Forgotten

I'd like to close this chapter with something about which I am both happy and proud. Many medical experts such as I, who are recognized as experts on a national and international scale, are often forgotten at home. I am honored to be an exception to this unwritten rule. Since 1973, when *Philadelphia Magazine* published the first in its article series, "The Superdoctors," I have been mentioned every year as a "Super Doc" in psychopharmacology. In 1973, only eight psychiatrists, including five from Penn, were mentioned. In 1994, this number had increased to fifty-five psychiatrists, including several from Penn who were mentioned under emeritus status (those who were spending less time with patients and more time teaching and writing). All emeritus psychiatrists, including me, were psychiatric leaders from Penn.

I was also honored in the book, *The Best Doctors in America, 1994-1995*. And more recently, in 2002, I was recognized by the Psychiatric Society of Pennsylvania with their *Lifetime Achievement Award*, which I accepted at a black tie dinner. Linda and all my family were with me to celebrate this great honor.

In 1995, I was honored by PENN with a portrait which hangs presently in the foyer of a large research building here at Penn, and in 2008, I received the *William Osler Patient-Oriented Research Award* from my own university in recognition of significant contributions to clinical research. In the announcement of this award, the committee stated that I was considered the world over as the "dean of psychopharmacology of anxiety disorders." Linda was not able to be with me that day, but was very proud of this recognition.

As I consider all the work I've done, I must conclude that if you are lucky and live long enough, you will eventually be recognized for your efforts.

Even at home.

10

Linda

As I reflect back on the past five decades, I am both inspired and humbled. But I can't close this book without dedicating a chapter to the greatest inspiration of my life, my wife of nearly forty-five years, Linda.

Ours was a uniquely beautiful and well-ordered relationship. In all of our married life, we divided our marital duties. Linda managed the checkbook, took care of our children, managed most of our social life, and selected the houses we lived in. I was allowed to vote independently, but for the president Linda selected. I was allowed to work, I was allowed to make all travel arrangements, and when in town, I tried to be home for our six o'clock evening dinner. This allowed me to work for a few hours more after the boys were in bed. And I really enjoyed being lovingly managed by Linda.

I was always reluctant to move. I never thought we could afford a new house, which may or may not have been true (remember, Linda managed the checkbook). Before we moved to our most recent home, about twenty-five years ago, I had turned down many houses that Linda and, in hindsight, I also had liked. Finally, Linda said, as she presented this final house for consideration, "Karl, that's it. I am moving. I hope you will, too."

I decided I would. And I have never regretted it. The home she had chosen became our dream house. By the way, I needn't have worried so much about whether or not we could afford the house. Linda paid the mortgage off not long after we moved in with the enormous profit she made selling the empty property behind our former house on Sweetbriar Road.

While Linda ran the house and the children, I still enjoyed lots of fun time with Steve and Mike. Larry was already out of the house by that time, at least during the school year.

From racing go-carts and riding on tractors to cleaning up the road behind our house when the boys were still very young, we had plenty of adventures. Linda always had the lemonade ready when we got home. In later years, it was tennis and golf. But Linda still did most of the organizing, carpooling, and providing the encouragement so we would stick with her arrangements for us. Every fall we would visit the Strasburg Rail Road and Dutch Wonderland in Lancaster County, Pennsylvania. I still do this today with my grandchildren.

Linda and I were always available to help our boys with their homework. And during homework time we tried not to have the TV on. One of our sons, I will not mention who, fought any change we recommended tooth and nail. I still remember that I once mistakenly made some edits to an essay with ink, and he rewrote the whole thing, not including any of my edits, being rightfully very upset with his father.

A few months after we moved into our Youngsford Road house, we acquired two puppies from a friend. Freddie was a yellow lab, and Shadow, a black lab. Freddie was Steve's dog, and Shadow was

Mike's. Freddie also had a soft spot in her heart for Linda. Whenever she left the house on some errand, Freddie always waited for her on the front lawn. The dogs were wonderful companions and lived with us for fifteen years. They died within two months of each other. At the same time we shared our lives with Freddie and Shadow, we also inherited an enormous cat, Kaiser. He appeared on our doorstep, having found his way to our house from the former owner's new house. Both of our dogs and Kaiser used a dog door, and so had the run of the property. Kaiser was an outdoor cat, and a few years later was run over by a car. We were greatly upset, and soon after installed an invisible fence around our two-and-a-half-acre property so the dogs would not suffer the same fate.

Before Freddie and Shadow, we had Scooter, an Airedale, who always brought me the morning paper. He also brought me other gifts, especially little animals, sometimes still alive. When our neighbor had kittens, some of them ended up at our front door, with Scooter sitting proudly next to them. After Scooter we had Nomie, a Siberian husky. Nomie liked to take mile-wide excursions and often came home in the dogcatcher truck. She was a lovely dog, but eventually we had to look for another home for her. My secretary's husband had finished veterinary school about that time and had settled in the country on a property perfect for Nomie—it had wide-open space. He offered Nomie a new home.

Shortly after we moved to Sweetbriar Road, Linda began the tradition of hosting a black tie New Year's Eve party for about forty friends, including The German Consul General and two of his staff and their wives, with whom we had become friends. The tradition continued for a number of years. The German consul and his family also spent several Christmas Eves with us, always bringing a cooked duck with them for dinner.

Velma, our maid and housekeeper, whose services we shared with friends when living at Scott Road, started to work full-time for us when we moved to Sweetbriar Road (we lived there for twenty years). She also moved with us later to Youngsford Road. Though Velma had half of one arm amputated, we hardly noticed. It certainly didn't affect her work. Velma came daily by bus, or sometimes was dropped off by one of her cousins. Velma also took care of the boys when Linda and I had to go on short trips.

Once, when we came home a day early from a trip, Steve stopped us at the top of our driveway so he could get rid of his friends, who were having a party at our house. Linda and I pretended not to notice. We needn't have worried anyway. Velma had everything under control. Velma was a wonderful person and was with us for more than thirty years until she retired. Velma and her sister owned a home in Philadelphia. For the whole time Velma worked for us, we made sure that she had Social Security for when she would be older, and we always made sure she had health insurance. After Velma retired, we still for many years kept contact with her at Christmas time. And we attended her seventy-fifth birthday, together with Steve, who was visiting at that time.

Larry

Linda was a great mother to Larry, whom she raised as an only child for the first seven years of our marriage, until Steve came along in 1971, and Mike in 1973. Larry spent each summer vacation with Crista's older sister, Ursula, her husband, Karl, and their four daughters in Germany, often camping on one of the German North Sea islands. During the years he was still in grade school, Larry talked in German in his sleep when he came home from his visits. When he was not assigned to an advanced English level in the next grade, Linda explained to the school that over summer vacation Larry spoke German exclusively, and thus naturally had to catch up with English. And, indeed after a few weeks, Larry always caught up. After completing elementary school, Larry went to the Haverford School for three years and then to the Lawrenceville School in New Jersey near Princeton for the last three years, the same school Linda's brothers had attended.

Larry studied at the University of Pennsylvania and the Free University of Berlin, graduating Phi Beta Kappa, and then went to graduate school at Princeton. Linda always accompanied Larry on his college trips, first helping him to select dormitory space and later, apartments. After Larry had received his PhD in German languages from Princeton, he taught for one year at the University of Cologne in Germany before he was offered a tenured professor position at the University of California in Santa Barbara. He has remained there all his academic life, and for a number of years as the chair of the German Department.

Linda helped Larry to choose the homes he bought in Santa Barbara. Later he moved to Hollywood and started to commute to Santa Barbara. He also teaches at an art college in Los Angeles, and in the summer, for the last few years, has been teaching at a private college in Saas Fees, Switzerland. With his portion of the money inherited from the sale of one of Linda's mother's beach houses, he bought a condo in Berlin's Hansa Viertel in the Tiergarten. Mike bought a cottage in the Endless Mountains in Eagles Mere, Pennsylvania, and Steve bought a condo and a bigger home way up in the mountains of Colorado.

As of this writing, Larry is now fifty-five years old and a bachelor. He is the author of many books and a beloved teacher. His class on vampirism drew more than one thousand students and had to be held in a movie theater instead of a lecture hall. Larry's well-attended lectures have been written up in national college guides for potential students as "must-attend classes." For at least a couple of years, Larry has also been a guest professor at New York University. I forgot to mention that since Larry uses psychoanalysis greatly in his literary work, he decided years ago to go through psychoanalytic training and become a California licensed psychoananlytic psychotherapist.

Steve

Steve, our middle child, was always our public service-oriented son. After graduation from Harriton High School, Steve spent the summer in the vacation town of Avalon, New Jersey, serving as a temporary policeman. Because he had to start his job the morning after graduation, he didn't even have time to go to the graduation party.

He joined the Gladwyne Volunteer Fire Company as a junior volunteer firefighter when he was sixteen. He drove an ambulance and was featured on a TV morning show, spraying water from the snorkel fire truck at the roof of Kiddy City, the site of one of the largest fires in our community. Since Steve was not yet eighteen, he couldn't enter burning buildings, and thus was the fireman every TV station photographed.

On his first visit home from college, Steve surprised Linda and me with an earring in one of his ears. We both pretended not to notice it. We knew that he would soon visit his friends at the Gladwyne Fire Company where he was still a member, and that he would be too embarrassed to go to the station with an earring. And, as we had expected, shortly after his arrival home the earring disappeared.

Only several years later did we learn from Steve how surprised he was at us that we had not responded as he had expected, namely, being upset and angry.

Steve graduated Magna Cum Laude from La Salle University with a major in criminal justice. He always wanted to join the United States Secret Service, and to get experience for such a position he applied to several police departments. He decided to take a job with the police department in Lakewood, Colorado, as this was one of only four departments in the nation that demanded a college degree.

Linda went with Steve to offer moral support for the interview and later helped him find his first apartment. After a few years with the Lakewood Police, Steve applied and was chosen for the Secret Service. After completing almost nine months of training, he served as a special agent with the Secret Service for four years protecting the president of the United States, vice presidents and their families, and almost all of the living ex-presidents and their wives. He met his wife, Heidi, while he was protecting the president of Rwanda, who was speaking at the University of Denver as a guest of a non-profit, humanitarian relief agency. Heidi was the communications director, and was arranging the event logistics, and the two had to work together for several days.

After Steve married Heidi in 2006 in Colorado Springs, Linda and I now had a second daughter. What a joy for the both of us. When expecting their first baby, Steve retired early from the Secret Service and rejoined the Lakewood Police Department, on the urging of his former division chief, who also encouraged Steve to try at once for sergeant, which he did. Steve enjoys being a detective sergeant overseeing the crimes-against-children unit; he is a great leader and is well-respected by the Lakewood police leadership.

Mike

Michael, or Mike, our youngest son, attended Episcopal Academy, serving as the president of his class for the last four years. He was a math major at Colgate University, which now comes in handy in his research of diabetes and endocrinology. At his introduction into Phi Beta Kappa in his junior year, Mike was the only student who did not praise his academic program when being asked what he liked about Colgate. Instead, Mike's response was "my fraternity," of which he was the president at the time.

Mike was the first to get married. He married his Colgate sweetheart, Alyssa, after one year of medical school at the University of Pennsylvania. The wedding was at Colgate. Mike is now one of the upcoming leaders at Penn, a great clinician, teacher, and researcher. Alyssa became the (first) daughter we'd never had.

I still remember attending a party given by close friends of ours not long after their wedding. My host and friend asked me to introduce Alyssa and Mike to one of the guests, and I blurted out, "Here is my daughter, Alyssa." I pointed over at Mike and continued, "They got married at Colgate." My friend responded, "But Karl, you don't have a daughter." Mike observed the whole interaction and merely smiled. Alyssa was so close to Linda's and my heart. And years later when Steve met Heidi and brought us another daughter, Linda and I felt like the happiest people in the world. We now had five children!

Linda the Real Estate Investor

Linda was a wise real estate investor. She bought our beach house in Avalon when Steve and Mike were babies and invested in several land properties in Telluride where we skied for many years. One particularly successful deal involved putting three downtown Telluride properties together, thus greatly enhancing their value. The money she made paid for all of our ski trips and much more. Her last deal was when she bought her mother's house in Vero Beach, renovated and enlarged it, and in 2004 sold it for a profit. Those profits, along with the profit from the sale of the beach house, provided us the funds to set up trusts for our boys and grandchildren.

Quite in contrast to Linda, I was a poor investor. When we sold the Scott Road house, after I had lived in it for six years, I only got the money out that I had put in. The same happened when I sold the ski-in, ski-out condo in Stowe, Vermont. And then there was the time I bought a race horse … that didn't even exist! The IRS pointed this scam out to me three years later. I had to return all my tax deductions and pay interest and a penalty, and still didn't get the money back that I had originally paid for the nonexistent horse.

Stowe and Skiing

The condo in Stowe might have been a poor real estate investment, but it turned out to be a wonderful family investment. The purchase was a bit of a snap decision. Linda and I had gone to a black tie ball downtown, one of the many charity balls Linda had me attend. Only when we arrived did I learn that it was the annual Ski Ball. We met friends of ours there. The husband told me he had just bought a ski condo in Stowe, after visiting there for several years, usually staying at the Inn of the Mountain. "You should buy a condo there, too," my friend said. "You will really enjoy it." Knowing my friend, a plastic surgeon, as a slightly compulsive, cautious planner, I bought a condo unseen the next day. And we never regretted it.

We went to Stowe every year, driving up on Christmas Day after exchanging our gifts Christmas Eve as they do in Germany. The drive would take between eight to ten hours, depending on the weather. We usually returned a few days after New Year's Day, depending on when school started again for the boys. Linda's mother, Bee, generously gave us cash gifts every Christmas. We used this money to hire the same private ski instructor, Bill, every Christmas we visited to help us improve our skiing skills and, most importantly, avoid the long lift lines. Larry, who often visited us over Christmas, never joined us in Stowe. He usually went to the Modern Language Association (MLA) meeting, held either in New York or Chicago at the end of the year. I am pretty sure Larry had given up skiing by that time anyway. Larry did, however, ski with me several times in Europe and Colorado when Steve and Mike were still too young to travel.

Each year we went to Stowe for a second time over President's Day Weekend, which meant taking the boys out of The Episcopal Academy for a few extra days. They didn't mind. We didn't sell the condo until the boys completed college, when we didn't use it anymore.

Despite my earlier mistake of taking Linda to the top of the mountain after only one lesson back when we were dating, she eventually took to skiing. She was an elegant, but cautious, skier and was a great sport in enjoying what her children and her husband liked to do. One year around Easter, I was in London and happened to read in the *International Herald Tribune* that a large, late-March snowfall was expected in Vermont. I called Linda, got on the next plane home, and we skied in early April. Linda enjoyed doing things on the spur of the moment.

Our ski season usually ended with a week of spring skiing, and later, after the boys were in college, with skiing over the New Year holiday in either the Rockies, Utah, or a few times with Linda only, in Europe. By the way, Linda, Larry, and I skied Vail the second season it was open. I still had wooden skies.

One year after Mike helped Steve move to Lakewood, Mike flew to meet up with Linda, Alyssa and two of her brothers, and me in Stowe. That was the year I was run over by a snowboarder on the slopes. Apparently, I was unconscious for a while, and finally skied down the slope to where everyone was waiting, all bloody in my face. We went to the physician in town who stitched up the wound in my head and rightfully told me to watch carefully for the next twenty-four hours for signs of brain damage. After we returned home, I saw a neurologist at Penn who, after giving me a few memory and cognitive tests, felt I had some impairment in these functions. He ordered an MRI, which showed a small subdural hematoma. Luckily it was gradually absorbed. Six weeks later, the follow-up MRI revealed I was completely normal. Thankfully, my minimal memory loss and cognitive damage had also disappeared.

Dedication, Wisdom, and Patience

Linda always had the best interests of her children in mind. When Steve and Mike were quite young, I agreed to be their soccer coach. Linda, without telling me, had signed me up for a training course to become a US Youth Soccer coach. The course met once a week for an entire winter at Lower Merion High School. The certificate I received still hangs on the wall in my office at the university with my medical certificates. When patients ask me about this certificate, I always tell them that it is the one I am most proud of.

The second time Linda signed me up for something was shortly after Steve and I went to the Philadelphia Boat Show. To everyone's surprise, including Linda's, I bought a speedboat for water skiing. I spent the next winter traveling, once weekly, to Conestoga High School for a boating course. I passed the final examination with flying colors, yet only Steve, who never took a boating course, was able to dock our boat in Avalon properly.

Linda was a patient saint. She put up with lots of my mistakes and not once in all of our married life did she get angry with me about them. Here are a few examples.

One day we were in the kitchen preparing to fly to Orlando for a meeting when a letter arrived from someone congratulating Linda and Mike for their birthdays. I didn't respond. I said to myself, "Oh, it can't be Mike's birthday today." I was right. It was Linda's, but that didn't register with me. She never mentioned anything about the fact that I had forgotten her birthday. After we arrived in our hotel in Orlando, Steve called us. I answered the phone and asked, "Steve, why are you calling?" He responded, "Naturally, to congratulate Mother on her birthday." That was the moment I recognized it was Linda's birthday. I quickly called two couples who were our friends, and who were also at the same hotel, to set up a birthday celebration dinner. And right after that, I ordered a cake.

During our last trip to London, we went to the Andrew Lloyd Webber show, *Lady in White*. I had not arranged for a limo to take us home, assuming that there would be many taxis. Well, there were lots of taxis, but they were all busy. As I stood in the shadows contemplating my mistake, Linda ran into the street, frantically waving for a taxi. A very nice taxi driver stopped. Only then did I come out of hiding. I was so embarrassed that I over-tipped the driver.

About ten years ago, on our trip to Amsterdam, St. Petersburg, and Copenhagen, I was using a new travel agent. She told me that

I didn't need a Russian visa. She was wrong. Apparently she'd only booked cruise ships to Russia, and when you stayed overnight on the ship, indeed you did not need a visa. Well, upon our arrival at the St. Petersburg airport, the border police took us into a special room, where (we can only assume) black marketers sold visas. It took more than three hours before we were finally able to receive a fax from our hotel, the Kempinsky, stating that we were their guests. This allowed us to obtain two visas, but not for the fifty dollars each that they would have cost at home, but for five hundred dollars instead. Linda sat there quietly the whole time, probably wondering when we would be taken to prison.

When arriving in Positano, Italy, a few years ago, we arrived in a terrible hotel. It was cold and had no heat. Again, I had tried out another travel agent. I was ready to take the limo back to Naples, Linda having not said one word, when I decided to call the Sirenuse hotel, the hotel into which our travel agent said she could not get us booked. Voila, there was an opening, and for five days Linda and I had the most wonderful time. Not surprisingly, when I had the concierge confirm our reservation at the Grand Hotel in Florence, which was our next stop, there was no reservation. But the concierge managed to get us in, nevertheless.

Linda signed me up several times as a chaperone for ski school trips over the weekend to Killington, Vermont. Just imagine, a ten-hour-long bus trip twice within two nights of sleep and two days of skiing. I still remember breaking my ribs on one of these trips, and I had to ski the next day full of painkillers. And I still recall the doctor's advice: "Do not catch a cold. Coughing will seriously hurt." I went on several of these trips, always having been signed up by Linda without consultation. And I enjoyed them all tremendously.

When asked about the main ingredient of our happy marriage, I always respond, "Linda was the ingredient." I usually add that Linda was also my best friend, but she was so much more. She was my *Lebens Gefaerte,* which roughly translated means "traveling companion through life, thick and thin, the good as well as the bad." Linda shared in my activities, and I in hers.

Shared Passions

Linda and I shared one other passion, namely, the protection of our Gladwyne community from excessive development. For a few years in the early 1980s, I made more headlines in the local papers leading the neighborhood opposition to the development of a life care facility in our midst than I did for my research at Penn. After more than two years, several hearings before the township Zoning Commission, multiple hearings before the Board of Commissioners, and a lawsuit that we won, a compromise was achieved.

The life care facility was eventually approved by our commissioners, after the requested density of eight units per acre was reduced to four units per acre. My public exposure led to becoming a director of the Gladwyne Civic Association, a position I left after a few years when Linda was elected director and chair of the zoning and building committee. During all this time we worked closely together on zoning issues, since we had become experts in this field. Linda spearheaded some of the zoning battles in the township.

Linda was always active in charitable work. Three organizations were particularly close to Linda's heart: The Gladwyne Library League, the Gladwyne Civic Association, and the various ladies' activities at the Philadelphia Country Club (PCC). Linda was chair of PCC Ladies Golf and, at another time, the Ladies Bridge groups. Linda also ran golf tournaments for cancer research and other important causes.

Linda was president of the Gladwyne Library League at a time
when the annual Library League cocktail party, held in the spring at
a private home, was the *dernier crie* of the Gladwyne social life. Husbands, including me, would cut their overseas business trips short
so that they could attend this party. The last time Linda and I were
at the League party was in May 2008, about six months before she
passed away. The *Main Line Times* had a spread on the party, and
among the several photos included was one of Linda and me. The
caption read, "Present at this year's annual cocktail party were Linda
Rickels, former president of the Library League, accompanied by
her husband, Dr. Karl Rickels." Linda was very proud of this, her
last photo in the newspaper.

Linda fought many battles for the Gladwyne Civic Association,
usually in front of the Board of Commissioners of Lower Merion
Township. When the children were attending the Episcopal Academy, Linda was active in the parent association, serving as chair-
woman of one of its balls, and also as president. There were many
other charitable events in which Linda enjoyed leadership roles. She
was involved in the Emergency Aid Society, the American Cancer
Society, the Scheie Eye Institute, the Ski Ball, and many other activities. Linda's photo frequently appeared on the society pages of the
Philadelphia and local papers. Sometimes she was standing with me,
but often those photos were of her with other prominent players.
In her world, I was always introduced as "Linda's husband." I loved
every minute of my role as her escort.

One of Linda's regular affairs was the annual cocktail party we
hosted at our house, held for our personal and professional friends.
This party got so large that we had to stagger the attendance. One
group of guests was invited from four o'clock to seven o'clock, and
another from six o'clock to nine o'clock. When our children were

older, they, their friends, and the friends' parents were always invited as well. For the years while the boys were in college, the party was always held over the Thanksgiving holiday. We liked to mix guests, be they professional or personal friends, young or old. When we stopped hosting this Thanksgiving party, many of our friends were disappointed.

Every Christmas time Linda would include a "Christmas letter" in her Christmas mailings to her family and friends. It would always be one page long, and would always start and end with short quotes or Christmas carol lines. The last Christmas letter Linda wrote was in 2007. I have included a copy in the photo insert.

Linda also liked to give luncheons for her lady friends, and she loved to throw baby showers or engagement showers for anyone she could think of. For years Linda would throw pool parties for my research group and, when the boys were still in high school, class pool parties for them as well. I had no skill at grilling, so we always had one of Linda's caterers take care of the food. I only had to take care of the bar.

Mike and Steve had many friends visit them at our house. But quite often, they never made it to the boys' rooms, because once they stopped to chat with Linda in the kitchen or at the breakfast table, they stayed. Sometimes they just wanted to enjoy a conversation, other times they came with concerns or personal problems. Linda was a good and quiet listener, doling out advice and guidance, but only if it was specifically asked for. She was there for everyone. More than once, girls who were friends of our boys ended up spending the night as our guests after a fight with their parents. Linda always helped these girls, but we always insisted that they let us call their parents and ask for permission for them to stay with us.

My father frequently told me, "Son, if someone does something good for you, you do something good in return. Don't just accept, but also give." Linda and I decided to follow this advice and to endow a chair in the Department of Psychiatry of the University of Pennsylvania in 1993 in my father's name. It was a thank you for the many opportunities the university had afforded me. In 1999 I endowed a second chair in Linda's name, for her unwavering support of my professional activities, which included spending summer vacations preparing NIMH grant applications, studying computer printouts at home while we watched TV, or spending time in Washington on study sections and/or chairing FDA committees.

I advised my children and grandchildren to "pick your battles, and select only those that you may have a chance to win." And I then asked which husband with his wife, or which child with his or her mother, had much chance to win their battles? I suggested that it would be much smarter to learn to say mostly, "yes, madam." This was a response with which I had plenty of experience. I used it often with Linda.

Vero Beach, Florida

In the spring of 1997, Linda's mother, who lived in Vero Beach on the east coast of Florida, decided to move into the Oak Harbor Life Care facility in Vero Beach, where she bought a lovely, two-bedroom, corner apartment. She offered to have Linda buy her house and that's what we did. Linda at once hired a builder, who, in early summer, as soon as the plans were drawn, started a renovation of the house that included tearing down the old kitchen and several walls to build a new one, including a breakfast room with fireplace and bar, which opened to a large family room. We then added a full addition including two bedrooms, two bathrooms, a hall, and a study. We also remodeled all the other rooms, put in new windows, and rebuilt the pool area. The builder told me that it would have been less expensive to tear the house down and build a completely new one. But we could not do this. It would have hurt Linda's mother.

We visited once in early fall during the building process, and in early January 1998, we drove by car down to Florida and moved into our house. The only furniture there was our bedroom furniture that had arrived one day earlier.

By the end of March we had most of the furniture for the house. Since I commuted several times to Philadelphia, Linda had to do much herself with a great interior designer. The designer showed Linda options, but Linda selected everything herself. For the next few winters, until 2003, we spent three months, from January to the end of March, in Vero Beach. Linda stayed the whole three months, and I commuted a few times between Vero and Philadelphia, yet did much of my work, including grant writing and working on books, in Vero. We kept one car in Florida, which I used to drive back and forth to the Orlando airport on my trips back and forth to Philadelphia.

In March of our first year in Florida, Linda hosted a large cocktail party at our house when our side tables were still mostly cardboard boxes instead of furniture. The party was a big success. In the year Steve graduated from the Secret Service Academy, Linda and I flew up to Washington D.C. for his graduation, and then took our Florida car, which he had borrowed, on the auto train back to Florida.

While in Vero Beach, we joined the Riomar Golf Club. It was situated on the ocean and its small membership of only two hundred members allowed us to play whenever we wanted to play without a tee time. Linda had many friends in Vero, and was actively involved in its social life, particularly in many golf and bridge activities, including tournaments. In many of these activities Linda's mother was also included.

After Linda got sick in December 2003, we only went to Vero one more time after she had completed her radiation treatment. During that short visit we sold our house, and this was the end of our Florida period.

Cancer

When I started this book, Linda was still with us. She left us in December 2008 for an infinitely better life than she had over the last six months here on this earth. I hoped to have this book completed while Linda was still alive, yet God had other plans. The book wouldn't be complete without telling you just a little bit about Linda's valiant five-year fight to overcome her illness.

Around Christmas, in 2003, Linda was diagnosed with an inoperable malignant brain tumor, a glioblastoma multiforme, located in the midbrain region. Her chances of living more than another year were slim. At that time the only symptom Linda had was a visual defect that she hoped to cure with new glasses. This was followed up with a visual field test and an MRI, which demonstrated a small, 2.5 cm tumor close to the thalamus in the midbrain. During the period when these tests were run, Linda still didn't expect anything serious, other than the need for new glasses. I suspected differently, but I kept my suspicions to myself, always hoping that I was wrong. After the MRI results were revealed, Linda also knew.

A brain biopsy confirmed the malignant diagnosis. Linda started at once with radiation therapy, followed by chemotherapy. She took a Temodar pill every evening for five days on a monthly schedule. This was combined with an antinausea medication to make it tolerable. MRIs were taken every two months to assess the treatment response. We knew that each MRI could reveal that the drug was not working, and with no other treatment available, that would mean a death sentence. What terrible stress and fear Linda must have been suffering during this time. It must have been almost unbearable. But Linda was very brave.

Our sons were wonderful. Larry and Steve visited several times while Linda was in radiation therapy, and Mike went with us to all the doctor visits, to the neurosurgeon, and the neuro-oncologist appointments. Mike also joined us when we went to Johns Hopkins for a consultation before Linda started treatment. Alyssa and the children were always there for Linda. Toward the end of Linda's illness, Heidi and Aiden joined them.

Shortly after the radiation therapy ended, Linda gave a luncheon at our house for all the friends who helped her during the radiation period and accompanied her to each treatment. What a wonderful human being Linda was. I don't think I would have even thought about such graciousness while in the midst of so much stress. But Linda did. Soon thereafter, and while Linda was still on chemotherapy, we flew down to Florida to arrange for selling our Florida house. Linda wanted to get closure with her affairs in this world, and I supported her.

Steve came down to visit us in Florida. I distinctly remember one particular incident while enjoying dinner together at a restaurant. Linda had temporarily lost some of her hair to radiation, and so she was wearing a scarf over her head. Apparently one guest at a neighboring table must have either looked at Linda or talked about her, because Steve suddenly got up, walked over to the other table, and gave the guest hell for his insensitivity and demanded an apology. Steve was always his mother's best protector.

Renovations and Remission

Soon after we returned to Gladwyne, Linda wanted to plan for the time she would not be in this world anymore to make it easier for the children and me. We first thought of moving to the Life Care facility in Waverly, but quickly rejected this idea. We then planned to buy the house next to Alyssa and Mike, which had just come available for sale. We hired an architect and were almost ready to go ahead, when we changed our minds. We didn't want to leave all our friends. We finally decided to build an addition on our house in Gladwyne, mainly so we could add an elevator. We loved that home so much. It held so many wonderful memories.

The renovations began in the summer of 2004. As always, Linda drew up the plans and had the greatest ideas. While the building was going on, Linda's chemotherapy seemed to work, and the tumor gradually became smaller. She stayed on chemotherapy for twenty-two months. By that time the tumor was no longer visible, and Linda's platelet count was greatly decreased as a side effect of the medication. Linda stopped therapy and for over two years her tumor was in remission. However, her visual defect and her fatigue stayed with her.

About eight months after the discovery of her brain tumor, Linda planned a large dinner party at the Philadelphia Country Club to celebrate four events. I give them here in the order Linda, not I, assigned them: first, my eightieth birthday; second, my fifty years in America; third, my fiftieth anniversary of being a psychiatrist; and fourth, our fortieth wedding anniversary. The party was a big success.

Linda was surrounded by all her family and friends and looked gorgeous. A disk jockey provided dance music and Linda danced with many of her children and friends.

I have never before shared the thought I am now sharing with you. At that party I couldn't help but think of the cocktail party I gave for Crista in honor of Ursula, Crista's sister, who had come to visit from Germany. Crista died six weeks after her cocktail party. Would the same happen to Linda? I was so afraid. I only hoped that Linda could not read my thoughts that evening. The very thought that Linda might have to leave this earth soon might well have been behind her desire to give the party. There are a few things in life that even in marriage one person might not want to share with his or her partner. I simply could neither talk about, nor accept, the possibility of Linda's early death. Of course, as we all know now, Linda was one of the very few with her type of brain tumor to whom the Lord granted five more years of life. We tried to savor and enjoy every moment of that time together.

I was so happy that even during Linda's illness we could still do many things together. In addition to visiting Positano on the Amalfi coast in Italy and Florence, we visited the Cotswold area of London, which Linda had always wanted to visit. From there we flew to her favorite city, Berlin. We also visited Berlin and Prague in 2006. And do not forget, Linda prepared for Steve's and Heidi's wedding in April 2006 and we made two trips to Colorado to prepare for the party Linda gave the night before the wedding.

In 2007, Linda and I took Andrew and Peter, our two oldest grandchildren, on a car trip to Williamsburg and Jamestown, towns we had visited many, many years ago with Gisela and Ahmad. Linda and the boys had so much fun. One day we drove to Busch Gardens, a large amusement park, and young Andrew persuaded me to ride a dangerous-looking roller coaster. And indeed, it truly felt dangerous to me. After we came off the ride, I saw the sign that read, "Dangerous for anyone over sixty-five years of age."

In the fall of the same year, we had American Express arrange a personal tour through China. It was one of our favorite trips. Sitting in our hotel in Beijing, we both admitted that this was such a good trip that we could have spent at least another week in China. And besides all these overseas trips, we had our children and grandchildren right here at home in Philadelphia and Colorado.

Some time before this trip, Linda had already stopped driving, mainly because of her visual defect, but also because of her constant fatigue. She had to give up golf at the beginning of her illness because of her visual field defect, and, therefore, focused more on her bridge game. She was on the first team of the PCC and continued to take advanced bridge lessons. Once a month on Fridays, Linda and I played mixed bridge at the club. This forced me to try to improve my somewhat limited bridge knowledge, which I did most evenings by studying my bridge books. We also regularly played bridge as couples. I enjoyed it very much. Linda was a good player, and played until she finally had to stop in August 2008 because of severe loss of memory and concentration ability. Friends would drive Linda to bridge, and I would pick her up at four o'clock in the afternoon at the club, combining it with a cocktail and an early dinner.

Recurrence

Just as in 2003, it was around Christmas time four years later when Linda's tumor recurred. The tumor was destroyed with a Gamma Knife, and this was followed up by more Temodar therapy. The tumor was kept under control for about six months. Then in August

2008, the tumor returned. A new treatment, Avastin, given via an intravenous drip, was initiated. Immediately, this affected Linda's platelet count and made her feel extremely weak. Avastin was eventually given a second time, and while the MRI showed that the tumor had gotten smaller, Linda's medical condition continued to deteriorate. She had lost all her strength and soon required a wheelchair to get around.

I will never forget one day in September 2008. Linda asked me to sit down with her at our breakfast table. She told me then that she had decided not to fight her illness any longer, and that she hoped that I would understand her decision. What could I do? I loved Linda. I could not fight her decision. But I had Linda promise me to hold off on her final decision until I had talked to our sons and we had seen our oncologist. All of our children and all three of Linda's physicians—her internist, her oncologist, as well as her neurosurgeon—accepted Linda's decision. Thus, finally, I also had to accept that she would leave me soon. Her doctors hoped that Linda would still be with us at Thanksgiving, but they weren't sure about Christmas. And, indeed, our whole family came together at Thanksgiving, and I had the Philadelphia Country Club cater the dinner. Linda sat at the head of the table surrounded by all her family.

Linda was cared for by some wonderful people Alyssa had found for us. Sarah, an acquaintance of Alyssa's, was with Mother during the day, from nine o'clock in the morning to four o'clock in the afternoon, most of her last year. I was always with her from four in the afternoon until the next morning, and every weekend. Toward the end I also had help in the evening from a nurse's helper. Since Linda had gotten ill, I had canceled all overnight meetings. So, when the fiftieth anniversary of the CINP arrived in July 2008, I did not want to go, but Linda insisted. While I was in Munich, Mike and his family moved into our house, Mike sleeping in the room with his mother during this time.

Alyssa and Mike were a great support to Linda. And Mike's children lifted their grandmother's spirits whenever they came to visit. The twins brought her small stuffed animals for comfort. And it was one of these little animals Linda held against her chest during the last few days of her life. Linda's illness, and eventually her passing away, must have been very stressful to her grandchildren. Nana, as her grandchildren called Linda, was loved by everyone. She simply did not have a bad bone in her body. Peter, then seven years old, observed and told me later that Nana would always control or correct me with just one word, "Kaaaarl."

For five years, my life was centered on Linda. I just couldn't accept that the time would come when we wouldn't be together. I tried everything to make her feel better, but I now know that I often was quite selfish. When Linda's condition started deteriorating, I did not want to accept it. I arranged for a personal trainer and for physical therapy, in the hope that Linda might grow stronger so she could continue to walk. I now know that I shouldn't have pushed her this much, particularly when she was ready to leave this world. But I knew, once Linda was in a wheelchair, that shortly thereafter she would leave me.

It has taken me a while to realize my selfishness. Linda was my strength, my love, and not only my wife and the mother of our children, she also was my best friend. I was afraid to live alone. How could I endure the days without her? We spent much of our time in our favorite room, our upstairs sitting room, and in the last two months Linda had her breakfast in bed, and I would sit next to her. It was so peaceful. At the end, Linda was at peace and prepared to go to heaven. She had so much to be thankful for. She was so happy that Mike and Steve brought two wonderful new daughters into the family. Mother was already ill when Steve and Heidi got married. But not only did both Linda and I attend their wedding at the Broadmoor Hotel in Colorado Springs, but Mother was able to give a great party the night before the wedding. And a few years later, Linda still could enjoy her fifth grandchild, Aiden, who is Heidi's and Steve's son. Linda was still able to hold Aiden in her arms that last Thanksgiving.

Linda passed away peacefully in my arms around seven-thirty in the morning on December 15, 2008, without any suffering. I now know that while I wasn't ready for Linda to leave me, Linda was ready to go. She had raised three wonderful boys who brought two wonderful daughters and five grandchildren into our lives, and Linda knew that she did not have to worry about me. She knew that I would continue my life, with her spirit all around me, and she would wait for me to join her in the afterlife when God was ready to call me.

As for now, I am content to continue working and spending time with my family. Almost every weekend one of my grandchildren spends a sleep-over with me. We play tennis and golf, go to the movies or watch movies at home, play chess or other games or computer games, and ping-pong. For dinner we usually go to a Japanese restaurant that my grandchildren call, "The Volcano."

Additionally, I have continued to travel with my family. Two summers ago I took Heidi, Steve, and little Aiden on a trip to Germany, first to visit with my sister, Gisela, and her family in Eschborn, near Frankfurt, and then to Berlin to show them the town I grew up in. This past summer I travelled with my oldest grandson, Andrew, to Greece, Italy, and Germany, retracing Greek and Roman history. Andrew had just spent the fifth grade studying Greek civilization, so the trip was particularly exciting for the both of us.

The coming summer it is my second oldest grandchild, Peter's, turn. And before that, Alyssa, Mike, and their children travel over Easter to Paris, and then on to my sister, Gisela's, family in Germany. Seeing the world with our children has always been an important part of Linda's and my life, and I think Linda would be glad that I am continuing this tradition with our children and grandchildren.

Someday I will have to leave this world. I hope I will be as ready as Linda was. I also hope to spend my final days in the same house where Linda and I had spent so many wonderful years. Just like Linda, I am so thankful for what great sons, daughters, and grandchildren we have. I have been fortunate to enjoy many professional achievements, too, and I know that life will move on in a happy and right direction for the loved ones I will someday leave behind.

Appendix 1: Family History

My Father's Maternal Ancestors

Bartholomaeus Bernhardi was born on August 24, 1487, in Feldkirch, Vorarlberg, Austria, and died on July 21, 1551. He was the Probst (head minister) of the protestant church Kemberg near Wittenberg. He studied at the University of Erfurt and Wittenberg and was ordained a Catholic priest in Chur, Switzerland. He converted to Protestantism and later married as a Lutheran minister in 1521. He returned to Wittenberg in 1512 where he was appointed professor of physics at a newly formed university. He defended his theological thesis in 1516, when Luther was one of the examiners. He became the dean of liberal arts and rector in 1518. He was the first Protestant rector of a university in Germany.

His son, Johannes Bernhardi, was born in 1522 and moved to Paderborn, Westphalia, as a Lutheran minister. Johannes' son, Bernhard Bernhardi, was born 1558 and later moved to Norden, Ost Friesland, to also become a Lutheran minister. His daughter was married to the chancellor of Graf (Duke) Enno III, who governed Ost Friesland from 1599-1625. Her daughter, Catharina Elsche, was married to Conrad Specht, a Lutheran minister at Aurich, all in Ost Friesland.

Conrad Specht died in 1645 while he was a Lutheran minister in Reepsholt. He was one of the first ministers to deliver sermons in High German. His son, Enno Specht, was born in 1632 and died in 1700. Enno's sixth child, Harm Specht, 1672-1724, became a master carpenter and married Grete Eden. Their son Conrad Specht, 1716-1786, became a carpenter and brewer. Conrad's son, Harms

Specht, 1754-1833, was a teacher. Harms' son, Diedrich Oltmanns Specht, 1796-1853, was carpenter and tavern owner in Reepsholt in Ost Friedland. His daughter, Ette Catharina (Specht) Harms, was born in 1833 in Reepsholt and died in 1908 in Sande. She was married to Harm Hinrich Harms, born in 1819.

Their daughter, Gesche Maria (Harms) Rickels, my grandmother, was born in 1866 in Helmste/Horsten, and married my grandfather, Johann Friedrich Rickels, in 1865. He died before I was born in 1922. My grandmother died in the late 1950s after I had already emmigrated to America. Thus, via my grandmother's ancestors, I can trace my roots back to a friend of Martin Luther, who started the Protestant movement.

My Father's Paternal Ancestors

The Rickels originally lived in Dithmarschen, a Marschland area in Holstein near Denmark, where they were farmers. In the late Middle Ages the farmers in this area formed a farmer-free state and only in 1559 were the kings of Denmark able to defeat them and make them their subjects. Finally in 1866, after the Prussian-Danish War, the land was returned to Prussia and combined with Schleswig-Holstein.

Gerd Hinrichs Rickels, 1785-1847, was born in Etzel, Ost Friesland. He was married to Gesche Rippen, 1793-1862, who was born in Marx. Their son, Gerd Hinrich Rickels, 1835-1905, was also born in Etzel and was married to Gretje Oltmanns, 1841-1918. Their son, my grandfather, Johann Friedrich Rickels, was born 1865 in Trettenburg, near Etzel and married to Gesche Maria Harms, my grandmother. He worked for the local postal service. He died in 1922.

My Mother's Maternal Ancestors

My great-great-grand parents were Johann Daniels, 1792-1866, who lived in Rheidt in the Rheinland, and Anna Christina Birmans, 1799-1867, who grew up in Alpen near Rheidt. My great-grand-parents were Friedrich Wilhelm Daniels, 1834-1883, who lived in Rheidt, and Johanna Sybilla Aldenhoff, 1838–1878. Their daughter, Maria Gertrud Daniels, 1866-1932, was my grandmother. The Daniels and Aldenhoffs owned small linen (primarily tablecloth) factories and tanneries. My entire mother's family was Roman Catholic. We still have a hand-stitched cloth with the name Aldenhoff on it.

My Mother's Paternal Ancestors

Johann Bernhard Roehrhoff, 1767-1836, was born in Buer, West-phalia, and was married to Anna Maria Genova Clant, 1754-1842, born in Kerschenbroich. He was the son of Bernhard Roehrhoff and Anna Katharina Kelle, and after leaving the family farm in Buer, Westphalia, took his inheritance and his horse and wagon across the Rhein to Willich. His son Anton Roehrhoff, 1801-1854, born in Willich, was married to Maria Christine Fliesgen, 1800-1880, who was born in Immerath. His son Johann Richard Roerhoff, 1835-1912, who lived in Willich, was married to Maria Katharina Thekla Flander, 1835-1869, who was born in Kempen. His son, my grand-father, was Anton Heinrich Roehrhoff, 1865-1931. He was married to Maria Gertrud Daniels, 1866-1932, and was a master blacksmith in Willich.

Appendix 2: Letter to Linda's Mother

Copy of letter dated November 24, 1963,
to Linda's mother, Bee Wilson.

Nov. 24, 1963

Dear Mrs. Wilson!

This will be somewhat of a rambling letter, yet I shall try to convey my thoughts to you as best as I can.

I realize that my love for Linda is difficult to accept by you. I certainly have many drawbacks, looking at me with your eyes, the eyes of Linda's mother. I am a widower, I have an almost nine-year-old son and I am seventeen years older than your daughter.

Believe me, I have searched myself and thought about Linda and me many, many times. When I came home from Europe, I honestly was not looking for anyone. I still had not been able to cope fully with Crista's death. And, parenthetically, during all the ten years of marriage, a very happy marriage, I never even looked at another woman. With all my possible faults, I am a "one woman" man.

Suddenly, when I met your daughter, everything changed.

Her loveliness, her warmth, her understanding, and everything else made me fall in love with Linda almost at once. I never for a minute thought about age differences at that time. Partly probably, because of my European background, which predisposes me for being less conforming than many of my American friends, I never look at age. We are still more romantic and believe in "feeling emotions," and have a smaller divorce rate than America. Marriage is not considered a "planned scientific" enterprise but a "joint venture" for life, founded on the basis of love and feeling and respect, and entered with the intention to "work on it."

I believe that in this respect, Linda's and my love has a much better chance than others to succeed.

Most of my friends in Germany have married girls who are ten to twenty years younger. My mother is eight years younger than my father, my friend's sister fifteen years younger, my other friend's wife sixteen years younger; even Kennedy was thirteen years older.

If one just looks around, even in America, one finds large age differences, and these marriages are usually very happy.

If I may say so, I may bring another "positive" aspect into a marriage. And that is that I have shown a capacity to lead a good marriage.

However, I agree, that for America at least, our marriage would be less conforming and conventional. But is this really bad? Don't Linda and I have to live our lives the way we plan it? And don't you think that a life based on love is better than a "cliché" life?

Advice can come from many sides, some is positive, some negative. But the one who gives "advice," and I speak here as a psychiatrist, never enters any risk. Only Linda and I will carry the responsibility for our future life. Finally, very often, the "advisor" advises because of his or her own problems and marriage deficiencies, and an advice becomes consequently nothing more than a personal bias and opinion of a troubled person without risk for them. Most of my friends just adore your daughter and support me whole heartedly. But two women, both older than I, both afraid of not only losing their looks but their husbands (husbands go their own way) in other words, both with poor marital adjustment and neurotic problems, advised me against Linda, and in fact tried to have me meet others, until I told them to go to "........."

Dear Mrs. Wilson, I love your daughter very much, and I am sure that I will be able to make Linda happy. Linda loves me too. Please trust us. Trust your daughter's and my judgments. It does not happen very often, and in fact it probably will never happen again, that Linda and I could love another person as much as we love each other. My love for your daughter is deep, pure, and honest. Please accept me!

May I close with a quotation from Goethe's "Hermann and Dorothea," pointing out the importance of doing what one thinks is right— irrespective of advice,

"For in these unsettled times, the man whose mind is unsettled only increases the evil and spreads it wider and wider, while the man of firm purpose builds a world of his liking."

Linda and I have a "firm purpose." Love will build a world of our liking. My mind is made up.

Please do not look at me as a "thief," I beg you.

Karl

PS. I was brought up to make my own decisions, because it is my destiny that I decide on. Linda and I have made our decision.

After concluding my letter to you, Mrs. Wilson, I remembered that you probably would like to know something about my background.

My father, just as his two brothers of whom one became mayor of a large German city and the other developed a large wholesale business, is a self-made man. He financed his own studies and has a PhD in economics; he was vice president, president, and co-owner in a larger German candy factory (600-800 workers).

We were bombed out during the war. The Russians nationalized the plant without compensation, my father started a new factory in West Germany, went bankrupt, and is now retired, writing poetry, and novels. He lost everything during and after the war.

My mother took up teaching again, after her children had grown up.

My sister (32) is an MD and is married to a Persian MD, both practicing in Frankfurt.

My brother (25) serves his internship and married last summer.

I grew up in Berlin, had many sports activities and, since I skipped a grade, I completed the Gymnasium at age seventeen, joining the German Army officers candidate school. I was with the Africa Corps in Africa, spent three years in America, and studied after the war in Germany.

We came to America in 1954 with $280. I trained in Iowa and here at Penn and decided to stay on. My financial situation is good, but I will never be a millionaire. Money for me is only a means to be used and not the final goal.

Money does not mean much to me. I was brought up affluently, I studied with nothing of my own but a little bike. I can live with money today and without tomorrow.

The only matter that counts is "emotional and marital happiness." Our heart is more important than our property.

Please understand me right. I will provide properly for us and our children. But I feel that the most important gifts that we can give to our children are:

a) to stand on their own feet,

b) to make their own decisions, never to shrink from responsibility and to stand to their beliefs, no matter what, and

c) love.

My note is longer than intended. I just hope you can understand.

Karl

Appendix 3: Advice of a Husband and Father to His Children and Grandchildren

- Happy and lasting marriage takes two people.
- Respect your spouse and what she/he stands for.
- Strive to be not only lovers, but also best friends.
- Make up before you go to sleep.
- Agree on the way you plan to raise your children.
- Teach by example and deeds, not only talk.
- Divide roles, and once done, respect the other's decisions.
- Be not only Dad or Mom, but also best friend and mentor.
- Once your children are grown up, advise them to find a job they like.
- A job you like and look forward to is more important than making money but hating your job.
- Be lucky to find and keep a good mentor to guide you.
- Have a positive outlook on life. Do not dwell on the negative. Shake it off and, if possible, learn from it.
- Choose your fights at home and at work sparingly.
- Sleep on it over night before making a hasty decision.
- Even in arguments and disagreements, always respect your adversary and his right to espouse his/her position.
- Learn from your mistakes.
- Be not afraid to make decisions—even wrong ones are better than none.
- Always be polite; politeness opens many doors in your life.
- And never regret to say, "I am sorry."

Notes

1. Hans Leip (poem and lyrics) and Norbert Schultze (Music),
   Lili Marlene, public domain.
2. Arnold Krammer, *Nazi Prisoners of War in America* (Chelsea,
   MI: Scarborough House Publishers, 1979).

About the Author

Dr. Karl Rickels is known throughout the world as the leading expert in the pharmacological treatment of anxiety disorders. He is the founder of the Mood and Anxiety Disorders Section at the University of Pennsylvania, professor of psychiatry, and the Stuart and Emily B.H. Mudd Professor of Human Behavior and Reproduction. As founder of the Penn program in the department of obstetrics and gynecology which treats and recognizes the special needs of women with mental health issues, his contributions continue to affect the lives of his many grateful patients. In 2008, the University of Pennsylvania awarded him the *William Osler Patient Oriented Research Award*, which recognized his outstanding achievement in patient-oriented research. He lives close to his family outside of Philadelphia where he is "Opa" to five grandchildren.